Home Care for the Client Who Has Had a CVA

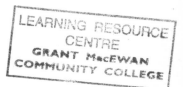

Home Care for the Client Who Has Had a CVA

Jetta Lee Fuzy, RN, MS
Director of Education and Training
Health Education, Incorporated
Fort Lauderdale, Florida

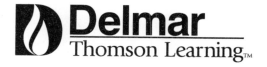

Africa • Australia • Canada • Denmark • Japan • Mexico • New Zealand • Philippines
Puerto Rico • Singapore • Spain • United Kingdom • United States

NOTICE TO THE READER

Delmar Staff:
Business Unit Director: William Brottmiller
Acquisitions Editor: Dawn Gerrain
Development Editor: Debra Flis
Project Editor: Stacey Prus

Production Coordinator: John Mickelbank
Art/Design Coordinator: Mary Colleen Liburdi
Cover Design: Brian J. Sullivan, Essinger Design Associates

COPYRIGHT ©2000
Delmar is a division of Thomson Learning. The Thomson Learning logo is a registered trademark use herein under license.

Printed in Canada
1 2 3 4 5 6 7 8 9 10 XXX 05 04 03 02 01 00

For more information, contact Delmar, 3 Columbia Circle, PO Box 15015, Albany, NY 12212-0515; or find us on the World Wide Web at http://www.delmar.com

Asia:
Thomson Learning
60 Albert Street, #15-01
Albert Complex
Singapore 189969
Tel: 65 336 6411
Fax: 65 336 7411

Japan:
Thomson Learning
Palaceside Building 5F
1-1-1 Hitotsubashi, Chiyoda-ku
Tokyo 100 0003 Japan
Tel: 813-5218 6544
Fax: 813 5218 6551

Australia/New Zealand:
Nelson/Thomson Learning
102 Dodds Street
South Melbourne, Victoria 3205
Australia
Tel: 61 39 685 4111
Fax: 61 39 685 4199

UK/Europe/Middle East:
Thomson Learning
Berkshire House
168-173 High Holborn
London
WC1V 7AA United Kingdom
Tel: 44 171 497 1422
Fax: 44 171 497 1426

Thomas Nelson & Sons LTD
Nelson House
Mayfield Road
Walton-on-Thames
KT 12 5PL United Kingdom
Tel: 44 1932 252111
Fax: 44 1932 246574

Latin America:
Thomson Learning
Seneca, 53
Colonia Polanco
11560 Mexico D.F. Mexico
Tel: 525-281-2906
Fax: 525-281-2656

Canada:
Nelson/Thomson Learning
1120 Birchmount Road
Scarborough, Ontario
Canada M1K 5G4
Tel: 416-752-9100
Fax: 416-752-8102

Spain:
Thomson Learning
Calle Magellanes, 25
28015-MADRID
ESPANA
Tel: 34 91 446 33 50
Fax: 34 91 445 62 18

International Headquarters:
Thomson Learning
International Division
290 Harbor Drive, 2nd Floor
Stamford, CT 06902-7477
Tel: 203-969-8700
Fax: 203: 969-8751

Library of Congress Cataloging-in-Publication Data

Fuzy, Jetta Lee
    Home care for the client who has had a CVA / Jetta Lee Fuzy.
       p.   cm.
    Includes index.
    ISBN 0-7668-0209-4
    1. Cerebrovascular disease--Patients--Home care.
    2. Cerebrovascular disease--Patients--Rehabilitation. I. Title.
      [DNLM: 1. Cerebrovascular Disorders--rehabilitation. 2. Home Care
Services. 3. Home Health Aides. WL 355 F998h 1999]
RC388.5.F89   1999
616.8'103--dc21
DNLM/DLC
for Library of Congress
                                    99-26641
                                     CIP

Table of Contents

Preface

As the home care aids (HCA) takes on more and more responsibility in home are, this expanding role includes participation in the recovery process of home care clients who have had a cerebrovascular accident (CVA). It is important for the HCA to understand this illness, become familiar with the equipment used, and the HCA's role in returning the client to the highest level of function.

This specialty training program has been designed to provide HCAs with training over and above their basic education and to give HCAs knowledge to prepare them to take care of these clients in a knowledgeable and supportive manner.

As more clients are discharged from rehabilitation centers and hospitals to the home environment, home care aides as assistants to the skilled nurse will be expected to play an active part as a member of the restorative team.

The specially trained HCA will understand the importance of caring for the client as a whole person, not just the body part that is weakened. The psychosocial, multicultural, and holistic aspects of each client must be considered in the care plan. Because many members of the home care team play a part, the HCA must be trained to understand each team member's role and function as the client progresses through the restorative process and into self-care.

In addition, the clients themselves and their families play an important role in the recovery process, and the HCA, as the client's advocate, can be influential in motivating and encouraging their valuable participation.

Whether providing the client with assistance in activities of daily living, ambulation, or exercise, the HCA with advanced training will no doubt spend valuable and skillful periods of time in the home.

CHAPTER ORGANIZATION

Short and concise chapters make this specialty module ideal as an in-service training resource. the module may be used in its entirely, or chapters may be spread across several training sessions. Chapter 1 reviews anatomy and physiology as it relates to clients who have had a CVA. Chapter 2 provides an overview of cerebral vascular accident, including the diagnosis, signs and symptoms, and treatment. Chapter 3 describes major physical losses associated with a CVA. Interdisciplinary teams and rehabilitation equipment are discussed in Chapter 4. Chapter 5 describes the rehabilitation/restorative phase. Chapter 6 reviews the basic roles and function of home care aides including observation and reporting, and documentation. Chapter 7 focuses on specially trained home care aides and the specific care they are expected to provide their clients including client care procedures. Client and family education, and the HCA's role, is discussed in Chapter 8. Basic safety and emergencies are discussed in Chapter 9. Chapter 10 defines the types of abuse and neglect, identifies possible signs of abuse, and discusses the HCA's role in reporting abuse. Chapter 11 describes psychosocial influences and how they affect the client's are.

FEATURES OF THE TRAINING MODULE

Helpful hints that emphasize key information the HCA should be aware of appear in each chapter of the module in gray shaded boxes in the margins. Key terms the HCA should know are bold-faced in the text and also included with their definitions in the margins. A case study is presented at the end of each chapter to provide the HCA practice integrating material learned in the chapter with clinical practice. Review questions are included at the end of each chapter to test the HCA's comprehension of the material learned.

ACKNOWLEDGMENTS

The author and Delmar would like to thank the following individuals for reviewing the manuscript and providing valuable suggestions:

Suellen T. Cirlli, RN, BSN
ORHS/Visiting Nurse Respite Education
Ocoee, Florida

Diana Hendon, RN, CRRN
Coordinator of Rehabilitation Nursing
Alacare Home Health Services, INc.
Birmingham, Alabama

Kathleen Lalley, RN
Clinical Supervisor
Yakima Valley Home Health
Toppenish, Washington

Kimberly A. Locker, MS, RN, CRRN
Nursing Education Manager
Sunnyview Hospital and Rehabilitation Center
Schenectady, New York

Introduction

The HCA who works as a specialist plays a vital role in home care today. He or she will become a great asset to the agency and to the clients they serve with this newly acquired knowledge.

The client who has had a CVA will be making great adjustments and experiencing serious losses, and the HCA's ability to assist them emotionally and physically will be rewarding. The HCA will be involved with other health care professionals who have dedicated their lives to assisting persons in creating a new life after this illness. The opportunity to work with these clients will bring health caregivers self-fulfillment as they have a great impact on these person's lives.

Returning the client to self-care is a long-term goal in all home health care situations. This is especially true of clients in a restorative program who have lost the ability to care for themselves as they once could. How much self-care is possible often depends on the client's motivation and the degree of brain damage involved. There is a big difference between returning the client with arthritis to self-care and that of a survivor of a brain injury. However, the main goal is for the health care team to determine the optimal level of self-care that can be obtained and then strive to meet that level, whatever it might be. Because every human being has the need to feel useful, caring for oneself must include some functions that the client considers useful.

Minimal self-care could simply be performing the activities of daily living for oneself such as feeding and bathing. At the other extreme, self-care could involve seeing a client who has had a stroke learn to drive a car again. Many clients who have had strokes go home from the hospital to lead normal lives through the rehabilitation process. Independence is a major factor and independence may simply mean performing ADLs or being back in the workplace and collecting a paycheck on a regular basis. The health care team must all agree on the plan and the goals, and discuss them with the client and family on an on-going basis. The client left with a chronic condition will have disabilities and needs which must be kept at a realistic level of rehabilitation during the course of the illness. Not only will the client recovering from a stroke have some residual effects, but also preventing another stroke is a very great priority. Therefore, the client may need to make lifestyle changes that could save his or her life.

Self-care deficits are common in clients who have had a stroke. Any of the clients afflicted with these losses may experience physical, emotional, and perceptual deficits. It is up to the physician and the therapist to determine if these deficits are permanent or temporary, and what measures should be taken to restore the client to an optimal level of function in view of these limitations.

The return to self-care must involve the physical, psychological, socioeconomic, spiritual, and environmental status of the client. The therapist and all the members of the team previously discussed must consider all five areas before a comprehensive self-care plan can be considered successful.

There are always going to be new treatments and devices to assist the client. It is the specially trained HCA's responsibility to keep abreast of these changes. These clients are disabled in that they have limitations in activity due to damage to their brain cells. With the specially trained staff, the client may alter their losses and the HCA may assist them through the process of being restored to a healthy level and a useful life through the rehabilitation process.

The key element to any restorative process is hope and motivation. The client also must have hope, hope that he or she will find renewed quality of life, and hope that tomorrow will be a day to look forward to because he or she will be a more active, independent, and healthy person. The HCA will play a major role in motivating the client who has had a stroke to use every day in an attempt to overcome the effects of the CVA.

List of Client Care Procedures

Anatomy and Physiology

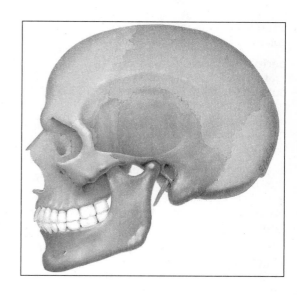

OBJECTIVES

Upon reading this chapter and completing the review questions, the home care aide should be able to:

1. Name the parts of the nervous system and describe the functions of the brain and spinal cord.

2. List the organs included in the urinary system and describe elimination.

3. List the organs included in the gastrointestinal (GI) system and describe elimination.

KEY TERMS

autonomic nervous system	elimination
central nervous system	neurons
cerebral arteries	peripheral nervous system

INTRODUCTION

To prepare HCAs to care for clients who have had a cerebral vascular accident (CVA) or a stroke, it is important for them to review the three body systems involved: the nervous system, the urinary system, and the gastrointestinal system. A basic understanding of the anatomy and physiology of each system will enable the HCA to understand the body and how it works.

NERVOUS SYSTEM

central nervous system that part of the nervous system that consists of the brain and spinal cord which coordinates the activity of the entire system by interpreting incoming sensory impulses and sending out corresponding motor impulses

peripheral nervous system that part of the nervous system outside the central nervous system and which consists of the cranial nerves, the spinal nerves, and the autonomic nervous system

autonomic nervous system that part of the nervous system which controls involuntary actions, and consists of the sympathetic and parasympathetic nervous systems

neurons any of the cells of the nervous system, also called nerve cells

The nervous system controls the activities of the body. It has three main parts: the **central nervous system** (which includes the brain and the spinal cord), the **peripheral nervous system** (which includes the cranial nerves and spinal nerves), and the **autonomic nervous system** (which includes the ganglia on either side of the spinal cord that control involuntary actions, such as heartbeat and breathing). The sensory organs—eyes, ears, nose, taste buds, and skin—are usually considered part of the nervous system.

The nervous system consists of nerve endings throughout all parts of the body and is made up of cells called **neurons**. Neurons are composed of a cell body, dendrites, a single axon, and end fibers (Figure 1–1). Neurons transmit messages through tissues, including nerve fibers and muscles. Nerve cells are much like electrical wires and have an insulating cover called the myelin sheath. When nerve cells are injured in the brain and spinal cord, they do not repair themselves and it is necessary for another part of the brain to take over the function of the part that was damaged. The rehabilitation process is necessary to help clients relearn activities after such injury or damage has occurred.

The brain is the most important organ of the body because it controls every action and reaction a person experiences. The brain is protected by bones (the cranium) and a cushion of fluid which also surrounds the spinal cord. Figures 1–2A and 1–2B show the brain and skull.

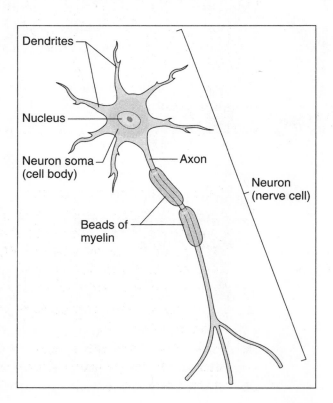

Figure 1–1 Structures of a neuron

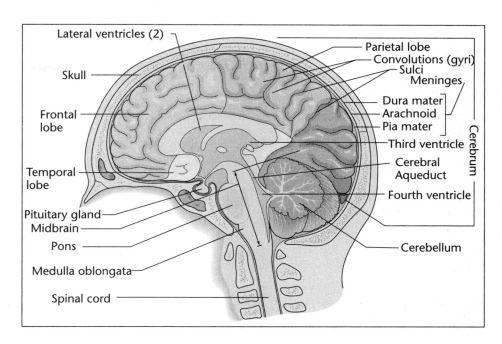

Figure 1–2A The central nervous system—brain and spinal cord

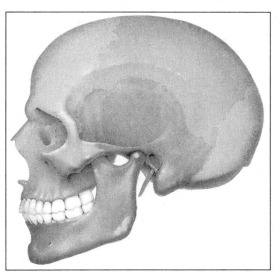

Figure 1–2B Lateral view of the skull

The brain has five main parts:

1. *Cerebrum* The cerebrum is divided into a right and left hemisphere. The right hemisphere controls the activity of the left side of the body and the left hemisphere controls the activity of the right side of the body. Some of its functions include thinking, memory, emotions, and reasoning.

2. *Cerebellum* The cerebellum coordinates muscular activity and balance.

3. *Pons* The pons is the base of the brain. The pons acts as a bridge whereby nerve cells cross to control the opposite side of the body.

4. *Medulla* The medulla is the pathway from the brain to the spinal cord. The medulla controls basic life functions, such as heartbeat, breathing, and digestion.

5. *Spinal Cord* The spinal cord contains 12 pairs of cranial nerves and 32 pairs of spinal nerves which branch to all parts of the body. The nerves act as highways through which the messages from the brain travel to the various parts of the body. Figure 1–3 shows the central and peripheral nervous system.

The brain and its functions are very complicated. The HCA who specializes in caring for clients with brain damage must understand that functions of the body are controlled by the nervous system by a unique pattern of messages which involve both voluntary (person controls the function) and involuntary (person does not control the function) methods.

The main arteries which nourish the cerebrum (**cerebral arteries**) are important to learn because the symptoms of a CVA are classified according to the artery affected. For example, the

- middle cerebral artery affects speech, vision, and muscles in the face and arms
- carotid artery affects numbness and weakness on one side, vision, headache, and speech

cerebral arteries any of the large vessels which carry oxygen to the cerebrum

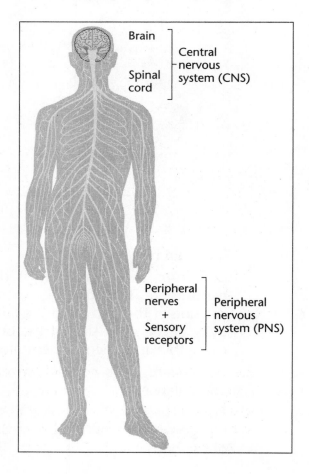

Figure 1–3 Central and peripheral nervous system

- verbebrobasilar artery affects weakness, numbness of lips and mouth, poor coordination, and slurred speech and dizziness
- anterior cerebral artery affects confusion, weakness, numbness of arm and leg, incontinence, loss of coordination, personality changes, and poor muscle motion
- posterior cerebral artery affects vision, poor sensation, coma, and blindness

It is important for the HCA to understand the brain and spinal cord function to better understand the body's reaction to injuries in these important organs. When a blockage occurs in a vessel from a blood clot, sufficient oxygen does not reach the brain and brain cells die, as does brain tissue. Because the cerebrum controls speech, sight, hearing, smell, and motor nerves, these senses are affected by the loss of brain cells in certain areas. Conscious thinking, or the ability to be awake and aware of actions and feeling, is diminished or lost in a person who has suffered a stroke. When motor areas are affected, the opposite side of the victim's body will be left weak or paralyzed.

URINARY AND GASTROINTESTINAL SYSTEMS

The urinary and gastrointestinal systems are important in the rehabilitation process because bowel and bladder training are often included in restoring the client to optimal function. The anatomy and physiology of these two systems will be limited to those areas involved in elimination.

The Urinary System

The urinary system is responsible for eliminating waste products through urine (Figure 1–4). These waste products result from burning food for energy. The urinary system is composed of the kidneys, ureters (the tubes leading from the kidneys to the bladder), the urinary bladder, and the urethra (the tube leading from the bladder to the outside of the body). The process of urinating is called **elimination**.

elimination the process of ridding liquid waste from the body; urination

After a stroke, the client may not be able to control urination. Early in the stroke, this may be due to mental confusion or loss of motor skills necessary to get to a bathroom or even to a bedside commode. In these cases, because of nerve damage, the bladder has a loss of sensation when filled with urine and the client does not feel the need to empty his or her bladder. In other cases, control of the urinary sphincter muscle is poor. This muscle tone usually does come back, but the bladder may go into frequent spasms, causing urinary problems. Urinary retention occurs when extensive neurological damage is not reversible.

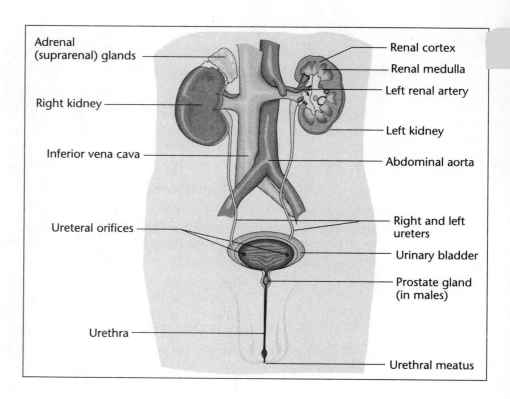

Adrenal (suprarenal) glands

Right kidney

Inferior vena cava

Ureteral orifices

Urethra

Renal cortex

Renal medulla

Left renal artery

Left kidney

Abdominal aorta

Right and left ureters

Urinary bladder

Prostate gland (in males)

Urethral meatus

Figure 1–4 The urinary system

The Gastrointestinal (GI) System

Elimination also includes waste matter from the bowels through the gastrointestinal system. The GI system breaks food down so it can be absorbed by the bloodstream and taken to body cells to be used for nutrition and energy. The GI system begins at the mouth and ends at the anus. It includes the mouth, pharynx, esophagus, stomach, small intestine, large intestine, and anus. Figure 1–5 shows the gastrointestinal system.

Elimination occurs through the rectum (the lower eight to ten inches of the colon or large intestine), and the anus (the body opening from the rectum). When neurological damage occurs in the bowel's sphincter muscle, bowel elimination problems may also occur. The client who has had a CVA will not have adequate motor skills at first to feed himself or herself and constipation or diarrhea may occur depending on the client's absorption of the type of foods offered. Lack of fluid intake also contributes to constipation. The lack of sensation or urge to have a bowel movement, coupled with the inability to express the need to move the bowels and poor motor skills to get to the commode, all contribute to problems with bowel accidents.

The client may also have a memory problem associated with elimination because voluntary muscle activities require not only sensation but also a step-by-step thinking process.

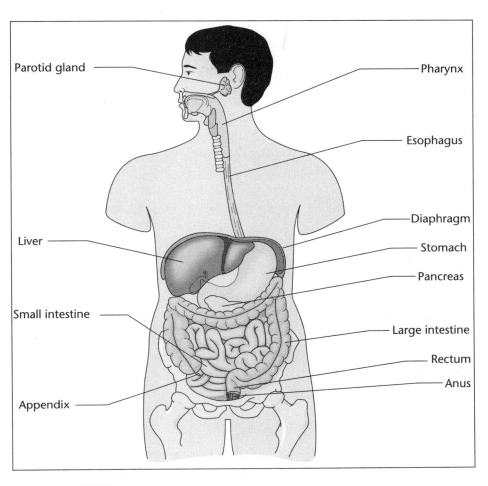

Parotid gland

Pharynx

Esophagus

Diaphragm

Stomach

Pancreas

Liver

Small intestine

Large intestine

Rectum

Anus

Appendix

Figure 1–5 The gastrointestinal system

SUMMARY

The nervous system is the system primarily affected in a person who has had a CVA. The cerebrum and its vessels are involved when there is brain cell damage, causing the client to have the symptoms related to a stroke. The urinary and gastrointestinal systems of the client are also affected as are the functions of elimination. The damaged cerebrum leaves the client with a loss of conscious thought and memory, and motor loss of the body side opposite the affected hemisphere.

CASE STUDY

Mr. Dunkin had a CVA three weeks ago. He is incontinent, and wears disposable briefs. This upsets him very much. The HCA finds him crying on entering his room. Mr. Dunkin tells the HCA he is crying because he thinks he will never get better, and will always have to wear a diaper. What should the HCA do?

REVIEW QUESTIONS

1. The three body systems affected by a stroke are the _____ system, the _____ system, and the _____ system.

2. The _____ is the most important organ of the body.

3. The spinal cord contains _____ pairs of cranial nerves and _____ pairs of spinal nerves.

4. Which of the following is *not* an example of an involuntary action?
   a. breathing
   b. heartbeat
   c. standing up
   d. blinking your eyes

5. Which of the following is a cerebral artery?
   a. aorta
   b. jugular
   c. carotid
   d. femoral

6. Which of the following is included in the GI system?
   a. bladder
   b. brain
   c. large intestine
   d. muscles

7. True or False? The spinal cord is part of the nervous system.

8. True or False? The middle cerebral artery affects incontinence and personality changes.

Match the system in the left column to its function in the right column:

9. _____ nervous system   a.   eliminates waste products

10. _____ urinary system   b.   breaks down food

11. _____ gastrointestinal system   c.   controls all functions of the body

12. Unscramble the following key term from the chapter: nusnreo _____

CHAPTER 2

Overview of a CVA

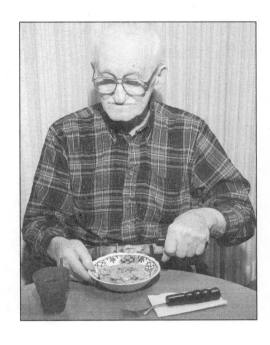

OBJECTIVES

Upon reading this chapter and completing the review questions, the home care aide should be able to:

1. List the risk factors of CVA and describe which of them may be controlled.
2. Describe a CVA including diagnosis, signs and symptoms, and treatment.
3. State the three phases of a stroke and how to recognize which phase the client is in.
4. Name the complications of strokes and list ways to prevent them.

KEY TERMS

aspiration

contractures

deformities

hemiparesis

hemiplegia

oxygen (O₂) therapy

semiprone position

spastic movement

window period

INTRODUCTION

Strokes are the number one cause of long-term disabilities in the United States. Because many families are affected by CVA, it is important for HCAs to specialize in the care of clients who have suffered a stroke. To begin any study of a disease, it is first important to understand it in terms of signs and symptoms, risk factors, diagnosis, treatment, and possible complications. It is also important for the HCA to look at the phases of the illness and learn how to prevent possible complications associated with it.

SIGNS AND SYMPTOMS

The five major signs of a stoke are:
1. Weakness or numbness.
2. Inability to speak or understand comments.
3. Sudden or intense headache.
4. Blurred or lost vision.
5. Dizziness or loss of coordination.

HCAs and other health care professionals should know these signs and symptoms and be ready to respond to them. Other signs and symptoms that could evidence a stroke include:

- severe headache or seizure
- change in mental state or loss of consciousness
- nausea and vomiting
- swallowing or speech loss
- one-sided paralysis or weakness
- possible eye disorders
- pulse and respiration increases
- hypertension (rise in blood pressure)
- elevated temperature

A transient ischemic attack (TIA) is a temporary loss of oxygenated blood to the brain and may be a warning sign of an impending stroke. TIAs may occur off and on, causing some mild neurological problems. Some last for minutes, others for hours, but all clear up in 12 to 24 hours. TIAs are reported in 50 to 80 percent of clients who have had previous CVAs. After the age of 50, the incidence of TIAs rises greatly. During a TIA, very small emboli (blood clots) cause blockages in small arterioles that create the classic difference between TIA and CVA: the return to normal function by the client. The signs and symptoms of TIA are similar to CVA and include double vision, slurring of speech, staggering or falling due to weakness of legs, and dizziness.

RISK FACTORS

Risk factors are factors present in the lifestyle of a person that increase the likelihood he or she will contract a particular disease.

Some risk factors can be controlled whereas others cannot. In the case of a stroke, the risk factors that cannot be controlled occur in those who are:

- male (higher incidence by 47 percent)
- African-American (incidence rate more than twice that of whites and Hispanics)
- female (longer life span and risk of CVA that doubles every decade after age 55)
- persons with Diabetes Mellitus
- persons with a history of prior stroke
- persons with a genetically high cholesterol level
- persons with a high normal red blood count
- persons with hypertension
- persons with parents or other family members who suffered a stroke
- persons with cardiovascular diseases

It is extremely important for the HCA and other health caregivers to understand the controllable risk factors of a stroke because it is the foundation of preventing strokes. The following are factors that are controllable to some extent:

- not smoking
- lowering and controlling high blood pressure
- treating and lowering high blood cholesterol levels
- treating high red blood cell counts
- avoiding oral contraceptives
- not being involved in alcohol and/or drug abuse, especially adolescents and young persons
- maintaining normal body weight

The following are lifestyle characteristics of persons who are at risk of stroke:

- smoking
- using drugs
- abusing alcohol
- being obese
- ignoring hypertension
- ignoring early warning signs

We will discuss prevention of stroke in more detail in the next chapter.

Nurses and physicians know that any sudden, excessive, or long-term fall in a person's blood pressure (BP) will cause a lack of blood supply to the cerebrum which may lead to stroke.

Situations such as shock, hemorrhage, surgery, certain diagnostic procedures, or medications may cause such a lowering of BP and these situations, because they cause high-risk, should be handled by professionally trained personnel. Strokes have long-term effects with mortality rates of 62 percent with a second stroke, and permanent disabilities devastating to those who survive. Knowing the risk factors and educating, not only clients but also the public at large, is the job of all health care workers.

DIAGNOSIS

The final diagnosis of stroke is done with blood tests, X rays, and careful physical assessment by the nurse and the physician. However, because early diagnosis at the time of an emergency situation is so important, the HCA should know what the American Red Cross' first aid course stated about recognizing a stroke and how to respond in the event of a suspected stroke.

According to the American Red Cross, the public should be taught the three *R*s of stroke:

1. *Reduce* stroke risk.
2. *Recognize* stroke symptoms.
3. *Respond* to stroke symptoms with an immediate call to 911.

There are some measures other than a physical assessment by the nurse or physician that may be done to diagnose a CVA. First, the five classic signs and symptoms of damage to brain function are almost always present in the acute phase (the first 48 to 72 hours). These include:

1. Loss of normal motor function on one side of the body.
2. Loss of speech.
3. Loss of vision.
4. Loss of normal mental function.
5. Loss of bladder function.

The tests that may be done to confirm a CVA include:

1. Skull X ray.
2. Computed tomography (CT).
3. Angiography (performed by injecting a contrast dye into the bloodstream and taking radiographic images to analyze the extent of the damage).
4. Magnetic resonance imaging (MRI) (imaging is done magnetically and the results show detailed pictures of the brain. This test takes up to one-and-one-half hours).
5. Electroencephalograph (EEG) (records the brain's electrical activity).

A physical, including careful neurological assessment, is still the most common way to diagnose a stroke. Nurses and physicians are taught to do careful assessments every time they treat the client. This confirms the diagnosis and documents physical changes as they occur. The HCA should also observe the client who has had a CVA on every visit to note changes that may be occurring, such as an improvement in the condition or a worsening, based on the signs and symptoms discussed. We will discuss observation skills in more detail in Chapter 6.

TREATMENT

Treatment or management of a client who has had a CVA depends on whether it is the acute phase (the first 48 to 72 hours), post-acute phase, or the recovery or rehabilitation phase (until maximum function is restored). In addition, new treatments are being offered in the emergency phase during the first few hours after brain attack occurs. These phases or time periods of a stroke are treated differently, but all are extremely important in the long-term recovery of the patient. Therefore, we will discuss each one separately.

Emergency Phase

The first one to three hours after the onset of stroke symptoms are a critical period. New "clot-busting" treatments using Activase® may restore circulation to the brain and increase the likelihood of patient recovery by one third with little or no disability. However, this treatment works best when given as early as possible and the **window period** (time frame in which the treatment will work) is limited. The Food and Drug Administration (FDA), the federal organization that approves all drugs before they go on the market, has approved the clot-busting drugs for ischemic stroke within the first three hours of symptoms. The new treatments do not work later in the course of the stroke, and recent studies show that 42 percent of persons with symptoms of stroke wait as long as 13 to 24 hours before getting help. Therefore, education is the key to early treatment.

window period the period of time in which a treatment or medical procedure will be of benefit to a client

Acute Phase

The acute phase is the first 48 to 72 hours after initial symptoms because cerebral edema reaches the highest level three to five days after cerebral thrombosis. Treatment of a stroke attempts to improve cerebral blood flow as much as possible. The following are medical ways to increase cerebral blood flow:

- improve oxygen levels in the brain by beginning **oxygen (O_2) therapy**

oxygen (O_2) therapy administering oxygen by means of a cannula, mask, or nasal catheter

semiprone position lying in bed with head and shoulders elevated

- giving medications that reduce edema, such as diuretics
- lowering cerebral pressure by placing patient in a **semiprone position** (about 30°)
- providing mechanical ventilation if stroke is life threatening
- watching for aspiration and pneumonia
- carefully monitoring and controlling blood pressure
- providing medication such as anticoagulants to prevent further thromboses
- reassuring the client who regains consciousness

Post-Acute Phase

The post-acute phase occurs after the first three days and before the client begins intensive rehabilitation. The post-acute phase is usually the time when the physician evaluates the client who has had a stroke to assess the damage that is reversible and that which is not. Sometimes it takes evaluations by therapists as well to determine how soon to start exercises and ambulation. There are physicians who specialize in physical medicine and rehabilitation. In very complicated cases, this specialist may be consulted to help establish a client plan during the post-acute phase.

Recovery or Rehabilitation Phase

Rehabilitation of a client who has had a stroke begins on the first day but is intensified after the critical first 72 hours and the assessment of the client in the post-acute phase. The HCA in the client's home may not care for clients in this early rehabilitation phase. It is important for all members of the health care team, however, to understand the treatment given to a client during all three phases as they interact and overlap, and there is no set time frame for any of the objectives of recovery.

During the first week, some treatment or management efforts are emphasized. When properly done, the restoration of body functions will be greatly improved in the long run. A hospital or rehabilitation center will most likely be the setting for the first one to three weeks of the recovery phase. The focus is on maintaining existing functions so no further losses occur, and the attempt to restore lost function by a coordinated effort of a team of health caregivers. This rehabilitation or restorative care will be discussed in detail in Chapter 5. The first weeks or immediate care in the hospital or rehabilitation center focuses on preventing complications.

COMPLICATIONS

A complication is an unexpected condition that occurs due to an illness or injury and which makes the recovery more difficult. The most important learning activity for HCAs is how to prevent complications whenever possible. There are complications of a CVA that may be prevented with proper care and management. Table 2–1 is an overview of the six typical complications experienced by a client who has had a CVA, and the preventions and treatments of each.

Contractures and Deformities

Contractures are a permanent shortening or lengthening of a muscle due to spasms or paralysis. **Deformities** are misshapen or disfigured parts of the body as a result of an injury, disease, or birth. Both may occur as a result of a stroke where one side of the body is affected with **hemiparesis** or **hemiplegia**. The brain injury resulting from the stroke causes neurological effects to the client's body, particularly the musculoskeletal system in extensive loss of voluntary control over motor movements. During the first 48 hours after a stroke, the deep tendon reflexes that are paralyzed are flaccid (weak and drooping). However, after 48 hours, the affected muscles show involuntary sudden jerks and twitching movements (**spastic movement**). This is due to the resistance to passive movement of a limb (arm or leg) from damage to the brain. Contractures occur quickly when there is spasticity.

contractures occur when muscle tissue draws together or shortens because of spasm or paralysis (can be permanent or temporary)

deformities physical distortion of a body part

hemiparesis muscle spasms or weakness

hemiplegia paralysis on one side of the body

spastic movement an involuntary movement of muscle

Table 2–1 Complications: Prevention and Treatment

Complication	Prevention	Treatment
Deformities, Contractures, Foot drop	• Positioning • Use of devices such as hand rolls and splints • ROM exercises	• Continued positioning • Use of devices such as hand rolls and splints • ROM exercises
Skin breakdown (pressure sores)	• Turning and repositioning • Good skin care • Use of a turning sheet	• Wound care protocol • Turning and repositioning • Drug therapy • Family education
Nutritional deficiency	• Careful monitoring • Family education	• Family education • Nutritional therapy including IV feedings or a nasogastric feeding tube
Blood clots	• Careful monitoring and observation • Lowered blood pressure	• Anticoagulant therapy
Shoulder pain	• Proper movement or positioning • ROM (without pulling or lifting affected arm)	• Heat therapy • Pain medications
Pneumonia	• Deep breathing exercises • Turning and positioning	• Drug therapy

The physical therapist (PT) will prescribe the proper treatment for prevention of contractures. Usually a firm hand roll is ordered to prevent hand contractures. This should have a smooth surface because rough textures may trigger spasticity. Special boots or splints may be used for foot spasms (footboards and tight covers lead to increased foot spasms). Footboards are used later in the flaccid period to prevent foot drop and shortening of the heel tendons. A bed cradle keeps the covers off the feet and prevents further spasms and irritation. Range of Motion (ROM) exercises are ordered. The PT will give specific instructions to keep affected joints in a state of flexion, which decreases the angle between two bones.

Skin Breakdown

When clients do not have control over their movements and position changes, skin breakdown or pressure ulcers are likely to occur. Skin breakdown will be discussed in more detail in Chapter 7.

Nutritional Deficiency

Because a client who has had a CVA and who is in the acute phase or recovery phase has difficulty swallowing and often cannot feed himself or herself, nutritional deficiency is a possible complication. The nutritional needs of the client must be addressed from the first day of care. In the acute phase, the physician may order total parenteral nutrition (TPN) which is given in liquid form by means of a high-protein sterile solution directly into the vein. Another type of feeding directly into the vein is intravenous (IV) therapy which is not protein nutrient but liquid replacement of glucose, minerals, and medications. Nourishment may also be given by tube feeding, either through a gastric (stomach) tube through the nose to the stomach, or by means of a gastric tube inserted into the client's abdomen directly into the stomach. Tube feedings are a nursing function, but HCAs will record intake and output for their clients who are on tube feedings (Figures 2–1A and B).

Nutritional deficiency is a problem for any elderly client because of the factors mentioned, but in addition, clients who have had a stroke also have decreased senses of smell and taste as well as chewing and swallowing difficulties.

The signs of poor nutrition include:

- weight loss
- poor posture
- edema in the extremities
- swollen abdomen
- rough, dry, flaky skin

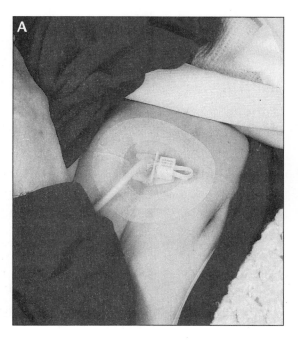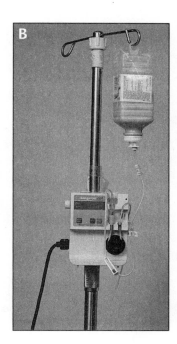

Figure 2–1 (A) Nourishment may be given through a tube inserted into the resident's stomach; (B) A pump automatically controls the amount of fluid, medication, or nourishment a client receives.

- dark circles under the eyes
- bleeding gums
- loss of ankle and knee reflexes
- thyroid enlargement

The client who has had a stroke should learn to feed himself or herself as quickly as possible to ensure that proper diet is returned as soon as possible. If the client is obese, or has high cholesterol or triglyceride levels, a weight-reduction diet may be ordered after restoration occurs. If the client has dysphagia, he or she should eat semisoft food and chew on the unaffected side. Foods can be pureed in a blender or mashed for easier chewing.

Feeding aids, such as adaptive plates and built-up utensils, may be used (Figures 2–2A and B). The following are suggestions to make eating easier:

- use special glasses and cups
- use unbreakable eating equipment
- use cups with weighted bases to prevent spills
- use cups with large handles or two handles
- use cups with lids
- cut a "V"-shape opening in a glass to prevent bending the neck
- use a straw to help drink liquids
- use a plate guard to keep the plate from sliding

Figure 2–2A The client feeds himself using a special cup and a foam-handled fork and spoon

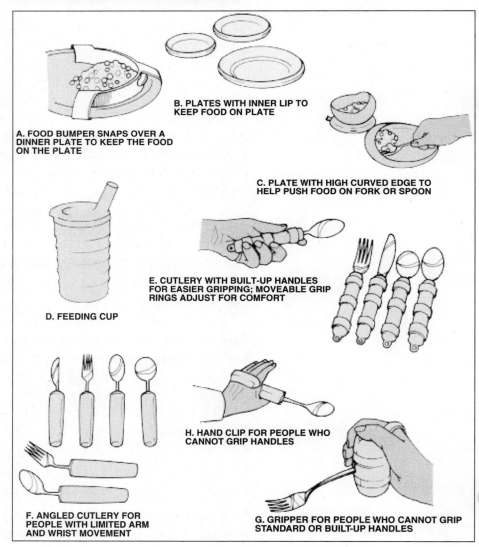

B. PLATES WITH INNER LIP TO KEEP FOOD ON PLATE

A. FOOD BUMPER SNAPS OVER A DINNER PLATE TO KEEP THE FOOD ON THE PLATE

C. PLATE WITH HIGH CURVED EDGE TO HELP PUSH FOOD ON FORK OR SPOON

E. CUTLERY WITH BUILT-UP HANDLES FOR EASIER GRIPPING; MOVEABLE GRIP RINGS ADJUST FOR COMFORT

D. FEEDING CUP

H. HAND CLIP FOR PEOPLE WHO CANNOT GRIP HANDLES

F. ANGLED CUTLERY FOR PEOPLE WITH LIMITED ARM AND WRIST MOVEMENT

G. GRIPPER FOR PEOPLE WHO CANNOT GRIP STANDARD OR BUILT-UP HANDLES

Figure 2–2B Special devices assist the elderly to feed themselves

Blood Clots

When a clotting disorder is the cause of the stroke, there is the risk of more clots that can block off the blood supply to other areas of the body. In addition, lack of activity increases the risk of blood clots.

Some preventative measures in the acute phase are turning, positioning, deep-breathing, and coughing exercises. Aspirin is commonly prescribed to prevent blood clots but HCAs and clients must be instructed to watch for:

- bruising
- hearing loss
- nausea, vomiting, or other GI problems
- small surface capillary bleeds on the skin
- bleeding gums
- stomach problems (aspirin should be taken with food or milk)
- swallowing problems

Chewable aspirin may be used. Other medications may be ordered to prevent clotting and the HCA should be alert for signs of bleeding or bruising. Clients who have had a CVA are encouraged to move as much as possible to improve circulation and rule out problems of inactivity, such as blood clots.

There are two forms of blood clots: a thrombus and an embolism. A thrombus is a blood clot that forms when deposits on artery walls cause platelets to form a clot. An embolism is a thrombus that breaks away and travels to another part of the body. During a stroke, the embolism travels to an artery in the brain and blocks the supply of blood to that area.

A second or third stroke while the client is recovering from the first may be fatal: therefore, clients must be watched closely and repositioned frequently in the acute and recovery phases.

Shoulder Pain

Up to 70 percent of clients who have had a CVA suffer from pain in their shoulders. This problem interferes with shoulder function, and restoring use of the arm becomes limited by the shoulder discomfort. There are three possible causes of shoulder pain in clients who have had a stroke including:

1. Painful shoulder from transfer injury.
2. Dislocation of shoulder from overstretching a paralyzed arm.
3. Shoulder-arm syndrome which includes swelling of the affected hand and a "frozen" shoulder.

These problems can be prevented by proper client transfers and positioning. Some physicians order the affected arm to be placed in a sling at first so it does not dangle and cause shoulder pain. ROM can also prevent painful shoulders and special exercises may be ordered to stretch the shoulder muscles.

Pneumonia

When clients are inactive for periods of time, they run the risk of developing pneumonia. The lungs do not expand and secretions and bacteria collect in the lungs, causing infection. Prevention includes positioning the client often and encouraging deep breaths. Once the lower lobes of the lungs develop pneumonia in an immobile client, it is difficult to reverse. Another cause of pneumonia in clients who have had a CVA is **aspiration** of food and liquids into the trachea and lungs instead of into the esophagus and stomach. Also, the client who has had a stroke may not expel sputum well, and aspiration can occur. The client should be encouraged to drink plenty of fluids and move around as much as possible.

aspiration the inhalation of food or fluids into the lungs

SUMMARY

The HCA who specializes in caring for clients who have had a CVA should first know the signs and symptoms, and the risk factors involved. The diagnosis is often determined by the five classic losses of brain function and by certain tests available to modern medicine. The treatment depends on the phase of the stroke from the emergency phase to the post-acute phase, and then to the recovery or rehabilitation phase. HCAs play an important role in the rehabilitation of their clients, especially in the prevention of complications which could affect the client's future ability to have a lifestyle in which the highest level of functioning is possible.

CASE STUDY

The client with high blood pressure complains of a severe headache, dizziness, and weakness in his or her left hand. What do you suspect and what action should you take?

REVIEW QUESTIONS

1. _____ _____ are factors that are present in a client's lifestyle that increases the likelihood of him or her contracting a particular disease.

2. The American Red Cross' three Rs of a stroke are:

   a.

   b.

   c.

3. The five signs of a stroke are:

   a.

   b.

   c.

   d.

   e.

4. MRI is M _____ R _____ I _____ .

5. EEG is E _____ E _____ G _____ .

6. Which of the following actions during client position changes may cause skin breakdown?
   a. pressure
   b. shearing
   c. friction
   d. all of the above

7. Which is *not* a way to prevent skin breakdown?
   a. massage surrounding area
   b. keep skin moist
   c. reposition frequently
   d. never rub skin dry

8. Footboards are not used early in the acute and post-acute phases because they:
   a. prevent shortening of heel tendons.
   b. prevent foot drop
   c. increase foot spasms
   d. not usually available

9. One-sided muscle spasms or muscle weakness is called:
    a. hemiplegia
    b. paralysis
    c. hemiparalysis
    d. hemiparesis
10. Spastic movements usually occur when in the client who has had a stroke?
    a. first 24 hours
    b. first 48 hours
    c. after 48 hours
    d. never
11. True or False? The post-acute phase of a stroke occurs after the first three days.
12. True or False? There are no physicians who specialize in rehabilitation.
13. True or False? The key to complications for clients who have suffered a stroke is prevention.
14. True or False? Rough, dry skin is a sign of poor nutrition.
15. Unscramble the following key term from the chapter: sutercatonrc _____ .

CHAPTER 3

Major Physical Losses Associated with Cerebrovascular Accident

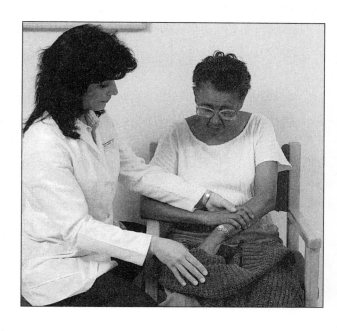

OBJECTIVES

Upon reading this chapter and completing the review questions, the home care aide should be able to:

1. State each of the five losses associated with a CVA.
2. Define goals of long-term recovery for each of the losses.
3. Demonstrate insight into a CVA case study.

KEY TERMS

biofeedback
cognitive loss
compensate

flaccid
incontinence

INTRODUCTION

There are many losses associated with a stroke, including emotional, financial, and job-related losses. Five major physical losses that occur in the course of a stroke that are common to all clients that the specially-trained HCA must consider include:

1. Motor loss.
2. Communication loss.
3. Visual perception loss.
4. Mental loss.
5. Elimination function loss.

We will look at each loss separately and discuss what each means in the long-term recovery of our client, Mrs. Brown. Mrs. Brown had a serious and massive cerebral vascular accident two-and-one-half-weeks ago involving the middle and anterior cerebral artery on the left side of the cerebrum. Her disabilities involve:

- speech
- vision
- facial paralysis
- right-side arm paralysis
- confusion
- right-side leg numbness and weakness
- bladder **incontinence**
- poor coordination
- personality changes
- poor muscle tone on the right side

The five main losses are all included in her status report and she is looking at a long, slow, and difficult recovery. Because each of these losses is going to affect her rehabilitation process differently, we will discuss each loss and what that will mean to Mrs. Brown personally.

> *Mrs. Brown is a 52-year-old mother of three children: a daughter aged ten and twin sons aged fifteen. She is a single mother, having been divorced for eight years. She is well educated, with a Masters Degree in education, and prior to this stroke, had an excellent job as an elementary school principle. Her income has been good and she has an extensive health insurance plan through the school system. Unfortunately, she does not have much in her savings account or in a retirement plan, and does not have long-term health insurance.*

incontinence the inability to control bladder or bowel function

MOTOR LOSS

Motor or movement loss is the result of damage to the motor neurons on one side of the body. Because upper motor neurons cross, the damage is evidenced on the opposite side from the brain damage (if the stroke occurs on the right side of the brain, the left side of the body is affected by motor loss). Terms frequently used to identify the location of a stroke are Left Hemi and Right Hemi, meaning that the left or right hemispheres of the brain are affected. HCAs should know on which side of the brain their client's stroke was located so they can approach them accordingly. For example, if the client was formerly a right-handed person and the stroke affected that side, the motor and other losses will have a greater effect on the client's recovery than if the left side had been affected. The client will have to overcome bigger challenges in dressing, feeding, writing, and even in ambulation (Figure 3–1). The HCA must understand that the frustration levels of the client who loses a dominant side are greater. The most common problem is hemiplegia or weakness on one side of the body. The recovery of this muscle function occurs slowly in some cases, beginning closest to the body and moving out to the fingers. Arm and leg recovery does not occur at the same time, and successful recovery of the function of one, such as the leg, does not necessarily mean the other will progress the same. Independence and regaining the motor loss is never ensured. Each loss is regained according to the brain's ability to recover from the damage. Poor outcomes in motor skills depend on some other indicators including:

- advanced age
- ability to understand commands
- memory ability
- previous heart problems
- other illness or chronic diseases, such as arthritis or diabetes

The client should be encouraged to use the uninvolved hand as much as possible, even at first, to assist the affected one. Functional electrical stimulation (FES) is a type of **biofeedback** (making unconscious body actions become controlled by conscious behavior) used in clients who have had a CVA to improve feeling and muscle contraction.

biofeedback a technique used to make involuntary actions of the body visible to the senses so as to make them voluntary

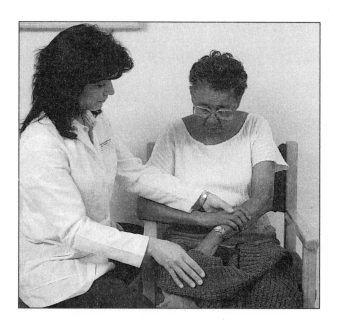

Figure 3–1   The resident who has had a stroke must be retrained in activities of daily living

To regain motor skills, the physical therapist teaches the client to use new skills and special equipment to compensate for lost functional abilities. The focus of PT for hemiplegia is on mobility and to strengthen major muscle groups both affected and unaffected by the hemiplegia. We will discuss PT approaches for clients who have had a stroke more fully in Chapter 4. As we discussed in Chapter 2, the early stage of a stroke is where the motor loss is seen in **flaccid** (no movement) paralysis and loss or decrease in deep tendon function. After 48 hours, increases are seen in the muscle tone as well as spasticity, evidenced by spasms or jerking movements of the arms or legs.

flaccid lacking normal firmness or stiffness

Mrs. Brown has had extensive right-side motor loss. Her right arm and hand were paralyzed for three days and are just beginning to settle down after almost a week of spasms. She is right-handed, and the loss of the use of that hand has been very difficult for her. She is using her left hand to move her right hand, and has a splint on the affected arm and hand to keep them in the proper position. Because of mental confusion, she forgets she has suffered a stroke, and in constantly trying to use her right hand, is always angry and frustrated at her situation. She is learning to use a walker, but it must be on wheels.

Her right leg is not paralyzed but is weak and numb. The previous muscle strength is not there and she is not nearly as coordinated as she once was. The resulting effect is that she limps when she tries to walk and she must now use the rolling walker to ambulate. The therapist believes Mrs. Brown eventually will progress to a cane when her right arm and leg regain strength.

She is at a disadvantage now because she is completely dependent on her health caregivers to assist her in moving about. She is thankful for the good nursing care she received in the past two weeks because she has no skin breakdown, no deformities, and no contractures.

COMMUNICATION LOSS

The greatest loss in communication in the client who has had a stroke is in language and the ability to speak. The four dysfunctions in communication are:

1. Dysarthria, difficulty in speaking caused by muscle paralysis.
2. Dysphasia, difficulty in speaking due to lack of coordination and inability to properly arrange words.
3. Aphasia, the loss of speech caused by loss of expression (see communication techniques in Figure 3–2).
4. Apraxia, loss of ability to perform an action which could be done before the stroke.

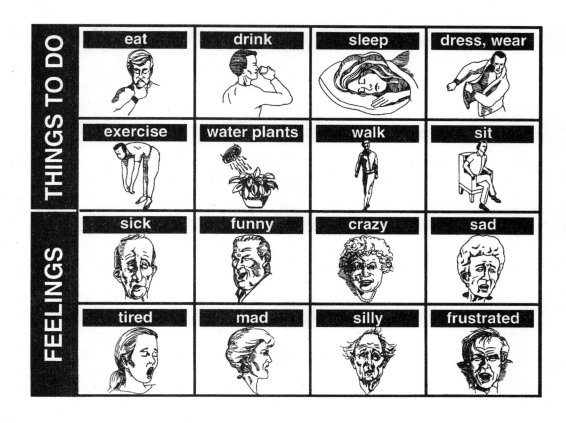

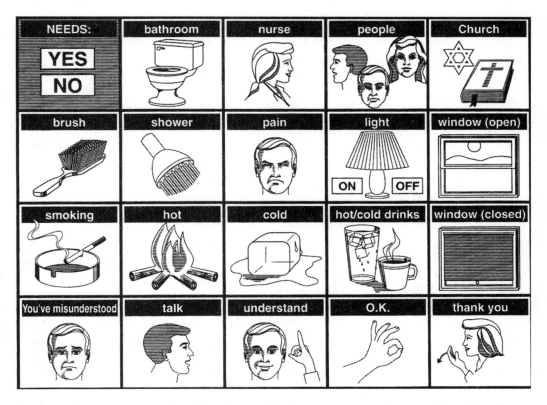

Figure 3–2 A communication board is often used to increase communication with a client who has aphasia

In dysphasia, the client's speech is affected, but usually he or she understands what is being verbalized by others. Aphasia is the most common communication loss in the client who has had a stroke. It may show itself in one of two situations: the client understands what is said but cannot verbalize a response; or the client cannot understand either spoken or written words.

General guidelines for communication with a client with aphasia are:

- a calm and supportive attitude
- touch, and a caring behavior to reassure the client
- eye contact
- slow and distinct speaking with a lower pitch and tone
- only one question asked at a time, and plenty of time allowed for responses
- visual aides, such as pictures, so the client can point to what he or she needs
- gestures, body language, and facial expressions used to communicate needs or wants
- speaking in short sentences
- attempting to fill in a word if the client is having trouble saying it

Early in a stroke, of all the five losses, communication is probably the one that frightens the client the most because there is the fear that another stroke will occur and he or she will not be able to seek help. The HCA should be sensitive to such communication fears and reassure the client that someone will always be nearby. Some communication tools other than speech may be helpful in keeping the client calmer, such as bells, buzzers, and even drums placed nearby in the early phases of the illness. Intercoms and alarm systems can be placed in the home to reassure the client. If there is a hearing loss, that should be evaluated and special telephones placed within reach. Hopefully, over a long period of time, the communication skills of reading, speech, and writing will return.

Mrs. Brown is a very attractive but overweight woman. Her inability to comb her hair or make herself look attractive is a problem, and not being able to ask others to do specific personal care tasks is the most difficult part for her. She tends to not want to bother her caregivers and lets her appearance take a back place at this time. Deep inside, Mrs. Brown is very discouraged but puts on an attitude of not caring about her appearance. It is easier not to try to speak at all than to slur speaking. She looks in the mirror and sees the right-sided droop of her facial muscles: she is sure she will always look like a monster. She has never been able to write with her left hand and refuses to try. Her children have created a communication system in which she can respond "yes" or "no" by blinking her eyes. Therefore, speech is unnecessary for her relationship with them at this time. But they look at her with so much sadness that their nonverbal communication says a lot to Mrs. Brown. She believes they are frightened about her recovery and the possibility of not having their mother back the way she used to be.

VISUAL PERCEPTION LOSS

Visual perception loss for a client who has had a stroke is caused by a disturbance between the eye and the visual cortex. This condition may be temporary or permanent, depending on the amount of damage. The affected side of vision is the same as the affected body side. The client sees only one side of the room or one half of the bed, and tends to turn his or her head away from the affected side. When the physician or nurse determines that one side of a client's vision is decreased, all staff, including the HCA, should be informed and adjustments made. Some specific adjustments for visual perception loss include:

- approaching the client from the unaffected side
- placing clocks, TVs, and the like on the unaffected side
- teaching the client to turn toward the affected side to attempt to compensate for the loss
- maintaining good lighting in the room

In clients with left-sided hemiplegia, there is often a loss of visual perception. This causes problems in dressing. The HCA should keep the client's room uncluttered and organized. The pace at which these clients work on self-care is slower than other clients who have had a stroke. The loss of touch is an additional factor in relearning skills. When visual perception loss is permanent, the client must be taught to compensate for the loss by looking from side to side.

Mrs. Brown's vision is improving every day, and the therapist and physician are very hopeful that a full visual recovery will take place. In the meantime, she keeps the room well lit and is getting good at turning her whole body to the right toward the person speaking to her.

MENTAL LOSSES

Frontal lobe brain damage affects high intellectual functions such as learning and memory. Some of the dysfunctions may be seen as:

- short attention span
- poor comprehension
- forgetfulness

- poor motivation
- increased frustration levels
- depression
- hostility
- poor cooperation

cognitive loss loss associated with thinking or reasoning

Cognitive loss affects every aspect of the client's life. When depression occurs, the client may cry more frequently than before, or desire to sleep all of the time. The restoration of thinking and mental losses occur gradually, as do the other losses. The client and family must, at some point, accept the fact that the client may never return to his or her previous cognitive ability. The loss may be permanent in some areas. In this situation, the client must be taught ways to **compensate**. For example, if the client always forgets to take medications, an alarm clock can be set to go off at the time as a reminder. Certain stimulation can trigger thinking and remembering such as signs, arrows, pictures, and music.

compensate find an alternate way of completing a task

Mrs. Brown's cognitive loss involves her ability to comprehend what is being said to her along with a very short memory span. Her short-term memory loss is a source of embarrassment and frustration for her. The therapists have assessed her loss and taken it into consideration in her rehabilitation plan. However, because of her previous above-average intelligence, the loss is extremely painful for her. She realizes some of the thought processes will return, but that more than likely, she will never be the same woman she once was in terms of intelligence, decision-making skills, and abilities of higher thinking processes. Just getting her brain to tell her arm and hand to work is exhausting at times. She cannot feed herself except with her left hand, so mealtime is a very messy experience. Her HCA has been providing her with pureed and soft foods which she can spoon and are easier for her to chew and swallow. Her dependency on IV nourishment only lasted for two days, but her feeding tube was in place for over a week and very uncomfortable in her nose. She is motivated not to have that form of feeding again and allows others to help feed her as she practices relearning this skill.

BLADDER INCONTINENCE

The loss of bladder control or urinary incontinence in a client who has had a stroke is due to several factors including:
- mental confusion
- inability to communicate needs
- impaired motor controls
- impaired sensation of bladder feeling
- loss of control of urinary sphincter muscle

Some of the muscle tone and deep tendon reflexes return in the client who has had a stroke, and bladder control improves. If incontinence continues after other functions have improved, the physician will know extensive and irreparable nerve damage has occurred. In some situations, bowel and bladder retraining may prove helpful (see Chapter 7 for the procedure on bowel and bladder retraining).

Mrs. Brown had a Foley® catheter in her bladder for a week because her bladder was affected by the stroke and elimination of urine was involuntary and out of her control. At this time, she is still incontinent of urine and must wear a disposable brief at all times. For Mrs. Brown, this is a devastating part of her recovery but she does not want to have an accident. She has even learned to change her own brief and is beginning to regain some sensation of her urinary sphincter muscle. Because her children do not know about this loss, and Mrs. Brown does not want them to know, she is very anxious to begin the bladder retraining program in a week or so. She says she would just die if her daughter saw her in a diaper.

Mrs. Brown's own mother, who is in her eighties, is in a nursing home completely incontinent and helpless. This is Mrs. Brown's greatest fear at this time. She is extremely depressed about the possibility of becoming helpless herself.

The client who must wear a disposable brief may find this a very embarrassing occurrence. One client may feel more strongly about one type of loss whereas another may not care at all. The client's culture and previous life will be a great factor in his or her adjustment to each of these losses. Regaining the ability to void independently may be a higher priority for some clients. This is a motivating factor in the success or failure of bowel and bladder retraining programs.

SUMMARY

All individuals who have had a CVA suffer the five major physical losses discussed in this chapter. Each client will differ in the degree of each loss and how he or she responds to these losses. The HCA who cares for these clients must be kept informed regarding each client and the status of his or her losses because each day is an important step in overcoming the changes and harm to the body associated with a stroke. Some of the losses may be recovered over time and the client must constantly be reminded of this by the HCA as care is being given.

CASE STUDY

The HCA arrives to care for the client recovering from a CVA to find him refusing to get out of bed and refusing care. He has aphasia and has been having great difficulty in communicating with his family and caregivers. What is the HCA's response to this client?

REVIEW QUESTIONS

1. State the five major losses associated with a CVA.

   a.

   b.

   c.

   d.

   e.

2. The loss of bladder or bowel function is called _____.

Match the following medical term to the correct definition:

3. Dysarthia _____   A. Difficulty speaking
4. Dysphasia _____   B. Loss of speech and expression
5. Aphasia _____   C. Loss of action ability
6. Aphraxia _____   D. Difficulty speaking due to muscle paralysis

7. True or False? Some clients never regain the losses discussed.
8. True or False? Motor loss is the greatest loss experienced by a client in the early stages who has had a CVA.
9. True or False? A loss of vision is always permanent.
10. Unscramble the following key term from the chapter: spocemaent _____

CHAPTER 4

Interdisciplinary Teams and Rehabilitation Equipment

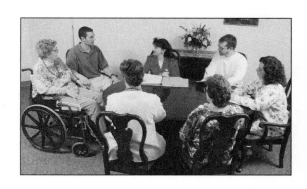

OBJECTIVES

Upon reading this chapter and completing the review questions, the home care aide should be able to:

1. Describe the difference between multidisciplinary and interdisciplinary teams.
2. Understand the HCA and PT care plans and the HCA and PT's role in each.
3. List the multidisciplinary members of the team and each one's role and function in the rehabilitation process.
4. State the goals and treatments of PT.
5. Describe adaptive equipment and their uses.
6. Describe personal care devices and their uses.
7. Describe safety devices and their uses.
8. Describe supportive devices and their uses.
9. Describe exercise equipment and their uses.

KEY TERMS

adaptive equipment

care plan

exercise equipment

interdisciplinary

medical social worker (MSW)

multidiscipline

occupation

occupational therapist (OT)

personal care devices

physical therapist (PT)

PT plan of care

rehabilitation center

rehabilitation equipment

respiratory therapist (RT)

safety devices

speech therapy (ST)

supportive devices

INTRODUCTION

Interdisciplinary two or more disciplines working together

multidiscipline various medical disciplines which make up a team to assist a particular client

An **interdisciplinary** team approach is usually used for hemiplegic rehabilitation. This team is more focused on specific client goals that are agreed on by the whole team, including client and family (Figure 4–1). The term **multidiscipline** is frequently used in other types of rehabilitation and refers to the different therapists (disciplines) included on the rehabilitation team. These include physical therapist, speech therapist, occupational therapist, respiratory therapist, and medical social worker. In a multidisciplinary team, each therapist sets his or her own client goals separately from the other disciplines.

For the interdisciplinary team method to be successful, communication must be excellent among the members. It is the key to the interdisciplinary process and function. The physician is usually the team leader with a skilled nurse case manager acting as coordinator for team functions. The team goals include:

- self-care in activities of daily living (ADLs)
- independent mobility
- psychosocial wellness
- some workable level of communication
- proper treatment program
- prevention of another CVA
- independence of client and family in decision-making

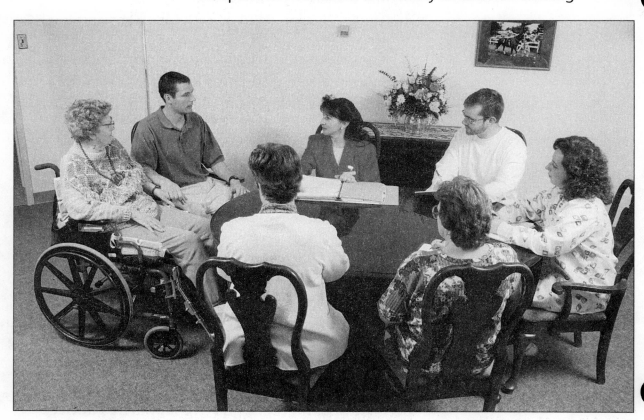

Figure 4–1 Residents and their families are members of the interdisciplinary health care team.

THE INTERDISCIPLINARY TEAM MEMBERS

The first function of the interdisciplinary team is to evaluate the functional level of the client assessments, both physical and verbal. When all have agreed on the client's status and restorative levels, client goals can be determined and the rehabilitation begin in earnest.

Physical Therapy

physical therapist (PT) uses exercises and treatments to increase mobility

The **physical therapist (PT)** is a health care professional who uses exercises and other treatments to help clients increase mobility. In clients who have had a CVA, there is also a focus on strengthening major muscle groups, which includes mobility in bed, mobility with a wheelchair, muscle strengthening for chair sitting, and gait training with assistive devices. Figure 4–2 shows a physical therapist helping the client increase mobility. The physical therapist is responsible for evaluating and treating clients

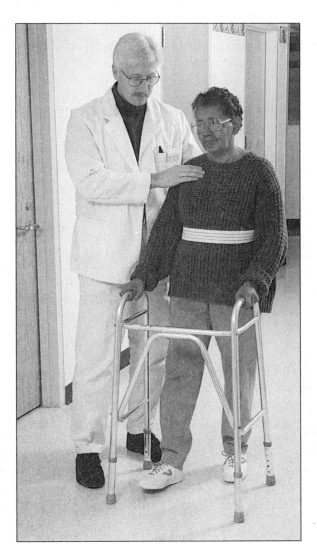

Figure 4–2 The physical therapist works to improve the resident's mobility.

care plan a plan instituted by the nurse or physician which contains the goals, instructions, and specific orders for a sick or injured client

with musculoskeletal and neuromuscular problems due to disease, injury, or developmental disabilities. In home care cases, the physical therapist is usually required to assess and evaluate the client, consult with the physician in developing a treatment plan, design a physical therapy **care plan** that other members of the team can utilize, and initiate and monitor the physical therapy treatments. There are physical therapy assistants who frequently do home visits after the plan is initiated.

Some of the treatment procedures used by physical therapists include:

- increasing strength, endurance, coordination, and range of motion
- stimulating motor activity to increase activities of daily living
- teaching the use of assistive devices
- attempting to relieve pain through prescribed therapy

In the case of a client who has had a CVA, the physical therapist will begin a program in the hospital that continues after discharge to the home. Some clients receive some of their PT as outpatients in **rehabilitation centers** if large pieces of equipment are required. Some examples include a client who requires parallel bars for support when learning to walk, whirlpools, kitchens and bathrooms setup for teaching proper use of wheelchairs, and large exercise equipment for strengthening muscles. Figure 4–3 shows the PT working with the client on the stairs at the rehabilitation center. Equipment in the home is usually smaller, and sometimes clients need a variety of both outpatient therapy and in-home therapy until they graduate to in-home therapy only.

rehabilitation centers provide outpatient PT when large equipment is needed

The goals of physical therapy in the rehabilitation phase involve the following:

1. Improving the quality of life for the client by returning him or her to the maximum level of functioning.
2. Increasing the client's productivity.
3. Offering a safe environment in the home with lowered risk of injury.
4. Decreasing pain.
5. Decreasing medications, particularly pain medications.
6. Promoting self-care and independence.
7. Increasing strength, flexibility, and endurance in light of the present disability.
8. Increasing self-esteem and emotional wellness.
9. Increasing day-to-day activities, both at work and at leisure.
10. Increasing the client/caregiver's confidence for discharge.

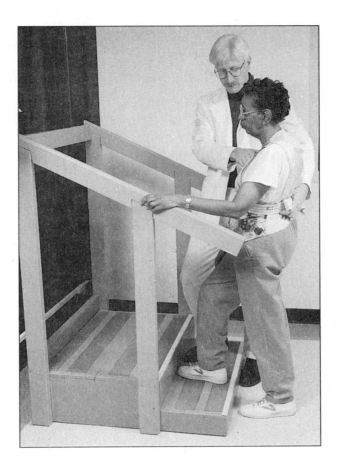

Figure 4–3 The physical therapist teaches the client how to use her body again and become strong after an accident or surgery.

Some of the restorative treatments in which the client may be involved are:

- therapeutic exercises
- transfer training
- gait training
- ultrasound
- electrotherapy
- prosthetic training
- muscle strengthening and flexibility exercises
- pain management
- traction
- massage

PT plan of care care plan specific to PT care and treatments

The physical therapist develops a **PT plan of care** which is reviewed by other members of the care team, including the HCA. The plan of care contains important information such as:

- client's diagnosis (onset or injury)
- level of functioning or functional limitations
- home environment appropriateness to rehabilitation
- equipment necessary

- any problems
- client goals
- anticipated rehabilitation potential
- discharge plans
- discharge date
- client's emotional and mental status
- role of other team members, including the family, client, nurse, and HCA.

"Therapists in home care cannot function in isolation. They must interact with nursing supervisors, staff nurses, and aides to coordinate care plans and ease integration of their services into the agency. . . . Changing perspectives demand that the whole team—client, physician, and all caregivers—develop the therapy program holistically."

(Hirn and Boin, p.11–12)

Occupational Therapy

occupational therapist (OT)
assists in restoring muscle coordination and strength by increasing the client's activity and independence

The **occupational therapist (OT)** is also a health care professional who provides rehabilitative services to persons who have had a stroke, persons with physical injuries, psychosocial problems, or developmental disabilities. Figure 4–4 shows an occupational therapist applying a splint. The occupational therapist helps clients restore muscle tone, coordination, and strength and assists with increasing activity to help the client become independent. The OT teaches the client to take part in his or her day-to-day care with such activities as personal care, eating, dressing,

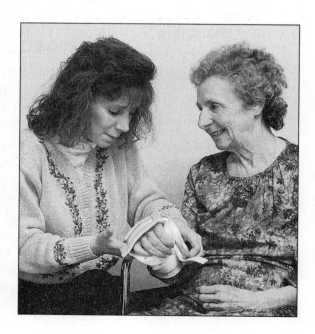

Figure 4–4   The occupational therapist applies a splint to the client's right arm.

Helpful Hint: In some cases, a PT or an OT Assistant may visit the client. The HCA may serve as the eyes and ears of the therapist as well as of the nurse.

occupation how the client is occupied in day-to-day living activities

Helpful Hint: In home care, the HCA may be supervised by a PT or an OT rather than the nurse if there is no nurse on the case.

speech therapist (ST) assists in speech and communication improvement

recreation, homemaking activities, and grooming. It is the OT's responsibility to establish a plan and monitor the client for the activities of daily living. A careful evaluation must be done and the OT and the PT usually work closely together to accomplish their goals. An OT care plan is also important, and the OT should include the HCA in assisting the client through the exercises documented in that plan. This is especially true in the area of setting goals and encouraging the client to participate in meeting the goals. The home often needs to be adapted to the client's disability and the OT is instrumental in accomplishing this task.

The difference between OT and PT is that occupational therapy applies all of the above treatments or procedures to help clients regain their *occupation*. **Occupation** refers not only to a person's work, but also how they are occupied in day-to-day living activities that include leisure and play activities. The following is a good example of the difference between PT and OT:

> Mrs. Smith has had a stroke with a severe disability and weakness in her left leg and arm causing functional limitation in walking. The physical therapist has been directed by the physician to teach Mrs. Smith to walk again, and to use specialized techniques to relearn self-care such as dressing, preparing meals, bathing, and caring for herself and her home. The two work together to restore Mrs. Smith to the highest possible level of functioning.

Speech Therapy

The **speech therapist (ST)** is a health care professional who assists the client to improve speech and communication. The client who has had a CVA with damage to the left side of the brain and who has difficulty with speech will find cotreatment sessions with ST, PT, and OT very effective. Clients who have a loss of speech have many psychological problems associated with difficulty communicating. The speech therapist must set up a long-term program to reteach clients to speak after strokes and other disabilities. This is a slow and painful process for both the client and the family, and the HCA, as a member of the team, can be very helpful in reinforcing the speech therapist's care plan. The speech therapist provides exercises and directions in the home for the family and other caregivers to incorporate into the daily plan. It is often the HCA's responsibility to oversee the practicing of these exercises. In addition, the ST evaluates the swallowing ability of the client to determine if special feeding and/or drinking techniques are necessary to keep the patient's nutrition at the highest possible level. In some cases, a registered dietitian may be called to consult on special diet orders.

Helpful Hint: Changes in speech, especially deterioration, should be reported because they may be signs of the disease process.

Some interdisciplinary learning activities are approached differently depending on which side of the brain the damage occurred because they have been proven to be different. The characteristics of the right- and left-side damage are shown in Table 4–1.

Respiratory Therapy

respiratory therapist (RT) restores the best level of breathing through exercises

The **respiratory therapist (RT)** is a specialist who restores the best possible level of breathing during rehabilitation. This includes having the client perform breathing exercises to increase lung capacity. As with any of the plans of care, the caregiver or the HCA should reinforce the exercises in order to enhance the rehabilitation process.

Medical Social Worker

medical social worker (MSW) deals with spiritual, economic, and psychosocial problems

The **medical social worker (MSW)** is the person who deals with the spiritual, economic, community resources, and psychosocial problems of the client during the rehabilitative process. Good communication between the MSW and the other members of the multidisciplinary team is vital to the success of the program (Figure 4–5). Depression is a common response to disabilities and can affect both the client's and the family's acceptance of the disability. The MSW assesses the psychosocial effects of the rehabilitation program and suggests actions to be taken to improve the situation.

REHABILITATION EQUIPMENT

rehabilitation equipment helps the client recover or improve activity

Rehabilitation equipment is equipment that helps the client recover or improve activity when a disability occurs. Assistive de-

Table 4–1	
Left-Side Damage	**Right-Side Damage**
Communication problems, learns best from demonstration	Visual-motor problems and lacks judgement
Activities to learn:	Activities to learn:
1. Transferring to/from a wheelchair	1. Break into small steps of instruction
2. Eating	2. Present material from affected side
3. Dressing using actual setting	3. Dressing using a pretend setting to lower stimulation
4. Verbal and nonverbal communication using facial expressions	4. Verbal and nonverbal communication use with no facial expressions
5. Gait training using demonstration	5. Gait training using practice

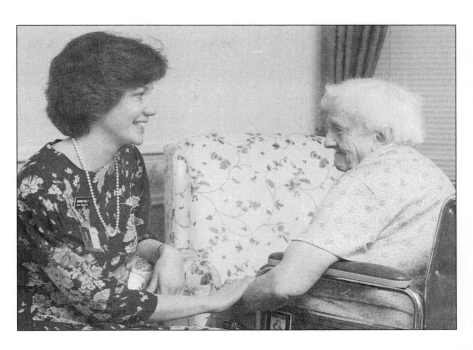

Figure 4–5 The medical social worker is concerned with the client's psychosocial needs.

vices are the most common pieces of equipment used in rehabilitation cases. There are five types of assistive devices:

1. adaptive equipment
2. personal care devices
3. safety devices
4. supportive devices
5. exercise equipment

Adaptive Equipment

adaptive equipment assists the client with ADLs

Adaptive equipment comprises those devices designed to assist the disabled client with his or her activities of daily living (Figure 4–6). Each item is designed to allow clients to perform activities they otherwise could not do. Figure 4–7 shows a client using adaptive equipment. Some adaptive devices are:

- aerosol can adapter which has a trigger to help the client hold down the nozzle
- plates with high edges
- cutlery with built up handles
- feeding cups with nonspill tops
- angled cutlery for people with limited arm motion
- long-handled tools for taking things from high shelves
- lowered tables and counters for wheelchair-bound clients
- one-handed knife
- food guard for the plate in order to keep food from spilling out
- hand clips for people who cannot grip handles

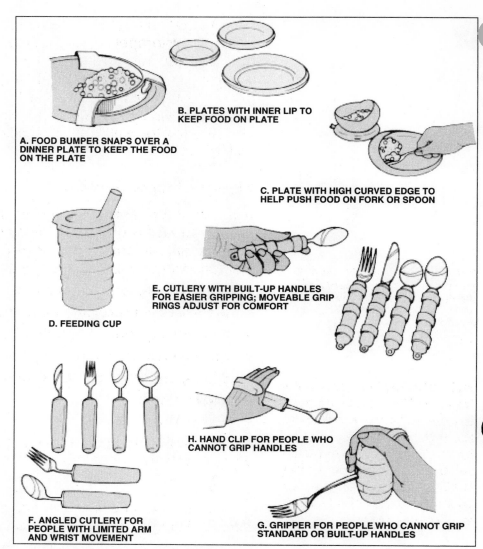

A. FOOD BUMPER SNAPS OVER A DINNER PLATE TO KEEP THE FOOD ON THE PLATE

B. PLATES WITH INNER LIP TO KEEP FOOD ON PLATE

C. PLATE WITH HIGH CURVED EDGE TO HELP PUSH FOOD ON FORK OR SPOON

D. FEEDING CUP

E. CUTLERY WITH BUILT-UP HANDLES FOR EASIER GRIPPING; MOVEABLE GRIP RINGS ADJUST FOR COMFORT

F. ANGLED CUTLERY FOR PEOPLE WITH LIMITED ARM AND WRIST MOVEMENT

G. GRIPPER FOR PEOPLE WHO CANNOT GRIP STANDARD OR BUILT-UP HANDLES

H. HAND CLIP FOR PEOPLE WHO CANNOT GRIP HANDLES

Figure 4–6 Special devices to help the elderly feed themselves.

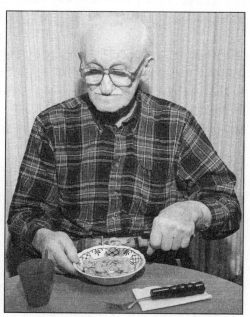

Figure 4–7 The client feeds himself using a special cup and a foam-handled fork and spoon.

A typical wheelchair for a hemiplegic client is usually one that is easily self-propelled and lightweight. It often has removable arm and leg rests and is lower to the floor than a standard wheelchair so the unaffected arm and leg can move it. The wheelchair should not be used by the client if ambulation with assistive devises is possible. A single-point cane may be all the client needs for walking. If a walker is needed, usually a rolling walker is best.

Personal Care Devices

It is very important that the clients in rehabilitation do as much for themselves as possible. This is especially true in personal care, and special equipment has been designed just for this purpose. The following is a list of some **personal care devices**:

personal care devices special equipment that is designed to encourage self-care

- long-handled brush and comb
- long-handled sponge for bathing
- nail-care equipment adapted for one-hand use
- grooming aids with built-up handles for easier grooming
- shoe grabbers and shoe horns with long handles
- dressing stick
- zipper aid
- stocking aid to help the client pull up stockings
- button loop
- trouser aid

Figures 4–8 and 4–9 show some examples of personal care devices. Figure 4–10 shows a client using a personal care device.

Helpful Hint: Sometimes it is faster for the HCA to perform the personal care activities than to allow clients to perform these activities themselves. However, remember that the goal is always for clients to reach the highest level of self-care possible.

Safety Devices

Because of the high risk of injury to clients who are unstable and have limited mobility, safety devices are an important part of the home setup during rehabilitation. The following is a list of some **safety devices** used in the home:

safety devices devices used to prevent accident or injury to a sick or disabled client

- locking wheels and side rails, as well as client call buttons, installed on beds
- whistles, bells, and intercoms for client reassurance when needing help
- locking guards on the wheels of wheelchairs for safe transfer (Figure 4–11)
- guard rails along corridor walls for assistance in walking
- strong banisters and extra rails along steps and stairways
- supportive rails in bathrooms for tubs, showers, and around commodes (Figure 4–12)

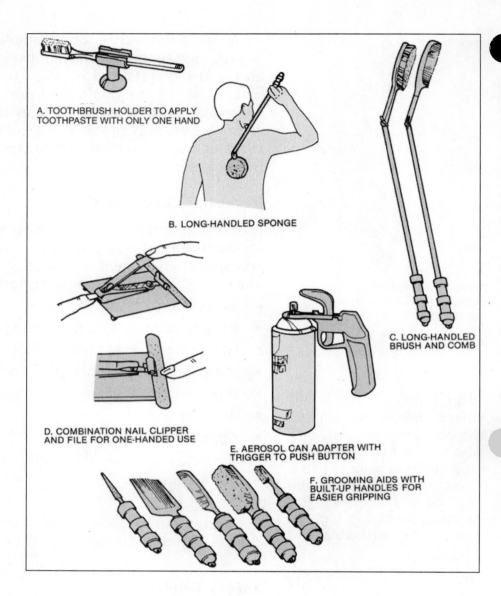

A. TOOTHBRUSH HOLDER TO APPLY TOOTHPASTE WITH ONLY ONE HAND

B. LONG-HANDLED SPONGE

C. LONG-HANDLED BRUSH AND COMB

D. COMBINATION NAIL CLIPPER AND FILE FOR ONE-HANDED USE

E. AEROSOL CAN ADAPTER WITH TRIGGER TO PUSH BUTTON

F. GROOMING AIDS WITH BUILT-UP HANDLES FOR EASIER GRIPPING

Figure 4–8 Personal care devices

- ramps built in the home to assist the client getting into and out of the house
- gait belts for supporting clients when ambulating (Figure 4–13)
- raised toilet seats (Figure 4–14)
- bath and shower seats (Figure 4–15)

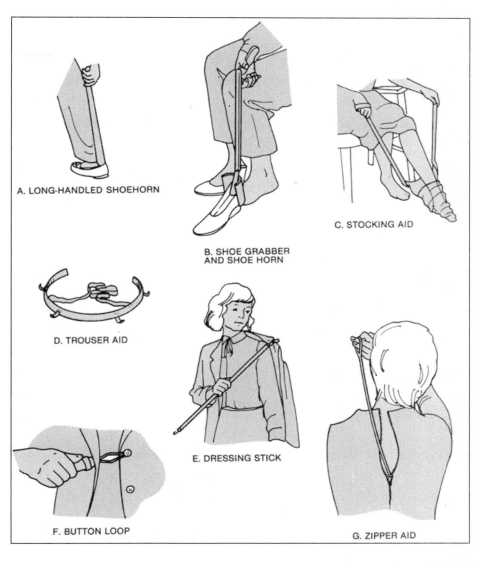

A. LONG-HANDLED SHOEHORN

B. SHOE GRABBER AND SHOE HORN

C. STOCKING AID

D. TROUSER AID

E. DRESSING STICK

F. BUTTON LOOP

G. ZIPPER AID

Figure 4–9   Adaptive devices for grooming and bathing

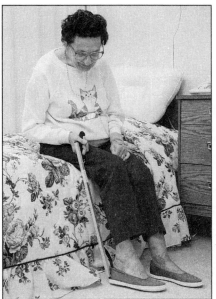

Figure 4–10   The client uses an assistive device to help her put on her shoe.

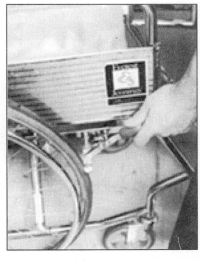

Figure 4–11   Always lock the wheels of the wheelchair before transferring the client to the chair.

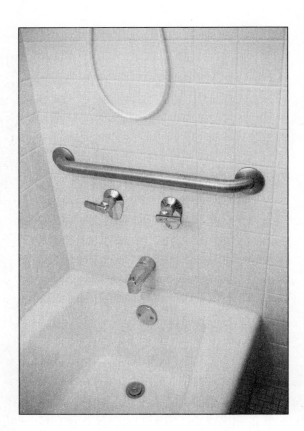

Figure 4–12 Safety features for the tub include grab bars and nonskid strips.

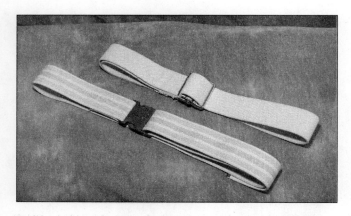

Figure 4–13 Gait belts or transfer belts are commonly used to ambulate or transfer a client.

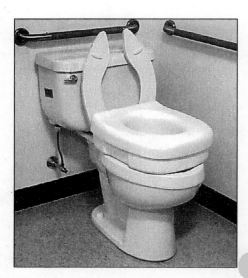

Figure 4–14 Raised portable toilet seats allow the client easier transfer onto and off of the toilet.

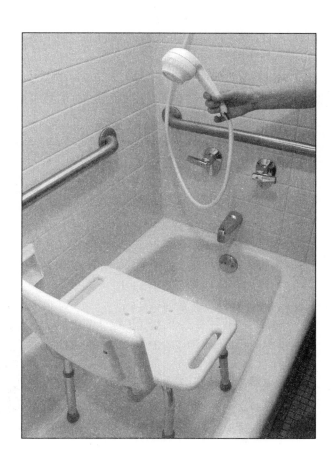

Figure 4–15 Bath chairs are often used to assist the client to get into and out of the bathtub safely.

supportive devices protect the client from falling when ambulating

Supportive Devices

Supportive devices are used to protect the client from falling when he or she is ambulating. The following is a list of some supportive devices:

- canes (quadcanes, blind canes, and seat canes)
- walkers
- crutches
- gait belts
- Hemi walkers
- seat walkers
- wheeled walkers
- wheelchairs and the numerous accessories available
- antitip wheelchairs

Figure 4–16 is an example of a supportive device used by a home care client.

Helpful Hint: The HCA must be familiar with safety and supportive devices to use them correctly as a role model for the client and family.

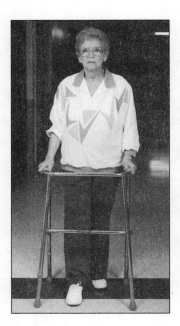

Figure 4–16 The client lifts the walker, places it in front of her, and then steps forward.

exercise equipment improves strength and mobility of the client

Exercise Equipment

Exercise is usually ordered by the physician and planned by the physical therapist or occupational therapist. However, the HCA should be familiar with the equipment used because he or she may be assisting the client with their exercises as prescribed. The following is a list of some **exercise equipment** used for rehabilitation:

- pulley devices used for arm and back strengthening exercises
- stretchable rubber strips to strengthen upper arms
- stationary bicycles for leg strengthening
- physioballs for hand-to-eye coordination
- exercise putty for hand strengthening
- leg weights and hand weights for strengthening of muscles during ambulation

The devices listed above are only a sample of the available equipment used in rehabilitation. The more complex equipment is ordered by a physician, the physical therapist, or the occupational therapist. If there is a piece of equipment in the home that you are not familiar with, ask your supervisor for a demonstration of how it is used. All equipment companies have excellent client education materials available for guiding the family and client, as well as the HCA, in its proper use. The safe use of all equipment can be ensured through a case conference with all of the caregivers present.

Helpful Hint: The HCA should never assist the client with exercises unless the therapist and/or nurse have included them on the HCA Care Plan.

SUMMARY

The members of the health care team who are involved in the rehabilitation process of the client who has had a stroke are all vital to the success of the recovery. This includes the specially trained HCA who should be informed as to the care plans and goals of the other team members including the nurse, physician, and other therapists. When special equipment and treatments are used to improve the quality of the client's life. HCAs must be knowledgeable enough to fulfill their role in restoring the client to the highest possible level of functioning. This chapter has covered many types of equipment and devices for such a purpose. When new ones come on the market, the successful aides will continue to study them so as to be able to best assist their clients in their day-to-day activities.

CASE STUDY

You are working in a rehabilitation center with clients who are recovering from CVAs. A new client arrives from a local hospital with crutches you have never seen before and you are assigned to assist her to ambulate with them. What should you do?

REVIEW QUESTIONS

Match the disciplines with the functions each performs in the rehabilitation process:

1. _____ Reteaches daily activities   a. PT
2. _____ Assesses mobility levels   b. OT
3. _____ Restores breathing   c. RT
4. _____ Reteaches speaking and communication   d. MSW
5. _____ Assists with psychosocial problems   e. ST
6. Bath and shower seats are an example of _____ _____ .
7. An example of exercise equipment is _____ .

8. What would *not* be included in the PT Plan of Care from the following list? (Check all those that apply.)

___ client goals

___ functional level

___ allergies

___ diet

___ emotional status

___ discharge plan

___ client's diagnosis

9. Which of the following is *not* an example of an assistive device?

a. pulley devices

b. wheelchair

c. overhead lighting

d. dressing stick

10. A long-handled sponge for bathing is an example of:

a. exercise equipment

b. supportive devices

c. personal care devices

d. adaptive equipment

11. True or False? All assistive devices are considered adaptive equipment.

12. True or False? The HCA should be familiar with assistive devices in order to help the client use them properly.

13. True or False? Hemiplegia clients using walkers do so first with walkers that roll.

14. True or False? Interdisciplinary and multidisciplinary are exactly the same.

15. Unscramble the following key term from this chapter: naidiceinrsiptrly _____

Rehabilitation/Restorative Phase

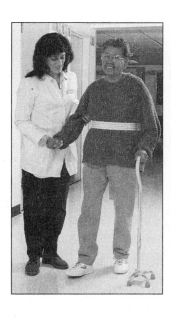

OBJECTIVES

Upon reading this chapter and completing the review questions, the home care aide should be able to:

1. Describe the importance of motivation in the rehabilitation phase.

2. Describe short- and long-term goals as they apply to the client who has had a CVA.

3. List the four main goals common to all clients who are in the rehabilitation phase.

4. State the ten steps of retraining for mobility.

5. List the activities of self-care.

KEY TERMS

compliance

expected outcome

mobility

motivation

nursing diagnosis

self-esteem

INTRODUCTION

Rehabilitation of the client who has had a CVA begins on the day of the stroke and continues until the client has reached the highest possible level of functioning. Sometimes this means returning

expected outcome the hoped-for results of short- and long-term goals

to the level before the stroke; more often it means attaining a level below the previous function. Either way, the client who has had a stroke goes through a long rehabilitation phase. For this phase to be a success, all the individuals on the health care team and the client and family must work together. If they have joined forces up to this point, the client's level of restoration is acceptable to everyone, and all involved are ready to set the goals for the **expected outcome** (the end result the client and team is hoping and planning to reach) of this final phase of care.

REHABILITATION PHASE

motivation act of encouraging another person to action

The client's mental state, including **motivation** (need or desire to do something) is toward reaching the goals and is of the utmost importance. This rehabilitation phase is a period of setting restorative goals (to get back or return to the former state of function). We mentioned that depression is always a possibility when a lifestyle has been severely changed, such as in these cases. The physician assesses the client's emotional level at this time in the recovery. After a stroke, the clients moods (state of mind) may change quickly, depending on the encouragement and support of the caregivers, especially the family. Anger is another emotion that may surface after a stroke. The HCA must remember that the client is not angry at the caregivers themselves, but rather at his or her own helplessness and the difficulty of the situation (Figure 5–1). In addition, the client is grieving for the losses experienced because of the illness. And the family and caregivers are grieving for the person their loved one was prior to the stroke. The health care team should try to understand that the client and family need to ventilate and talk about their feel-

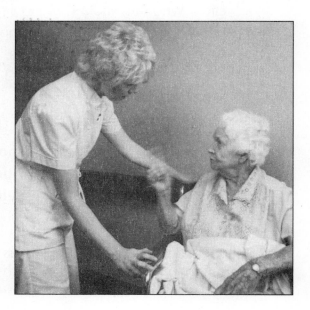

Figure 5–1 Clients may become frustrated with the changes occurring in their lives.

ings. They will learn to accept the final outcome, but it will be a slow and often emotionally painful experience.

The health care team, including the specially trained HCA, must keep the family and client focused on recovery because getting to the end result will be hard work for all involved.

Motivation

The most important aspect of caring for the client who has had a stroke in the rehabilitation phase is to keep him or her motivated. This requires much encouragement from all who influence the client, including the following important persons:

- himself or herself
- physician
- family
- HCAs
- nurses
- therapists
- clergy or spiritual leaders
- friends and neighbors

self-esteem self respect; self-image

Motivation of the client begins when all the negative feelings have been addressed. The client's **self-esteem** is critical to the acceptance of attempts by others to encourage and motivate him or her. Self-esteem is how a person feels about himself or herself. In the case of the client who has had a stroke, with all the losses we have discussed, the loss of self-esteem may be the most difficult with which to deal. Often, self-esteem is associated with independence which is, in the end, the greatest loss of all for human beings.

In our society, human strength is valued and weakness is feared. To lose one's independence or the ability to care completely for oneself is a great fear, especially among the elderly. When caring for clients who have had a stroke, the HCA must give them as much opportunity to be as independent as possible (Figure 5–2). This will increase their self-esteem and pave the way for others to motivate them to become as well as possible and to accept themselves at whatever level that is. This, of course, is easier said than done. Acceptance in the face of limitations and even a small loss of independence is often very difficult. Motivation involves meeting the clients' conscious and unconscious needs by using their interests and your rewards to encourage a positive attitude and behavior focused on personal and individual goals. How can the HCA caring for a client who has had a stoke motivate that person to keep pushing themselves every day until he or she reaches the goal of recovery? The first step, as we stated, is to build the client's self-esteem.

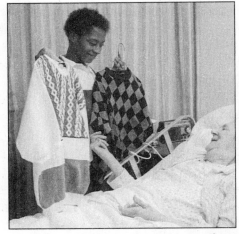

Figure 5–2 Whenever necessary, assist the resident but allow her to make her own decisions.

When attempting to motivate another person, it is important to invest time and effort into getting to know that person as an individual including likes and dislikes, interests, and expectations. There must be a bond between the person doing the motivating and the person being motivated or there is no basis for a relationship. Praise and credit are good motivational rewards for all individuals (Figure 5–3). We all like to think we can accomplish something worthwhile. In the case of the client who has had a stroke that may be something as simple as relearning the skills to dress himself or herself.

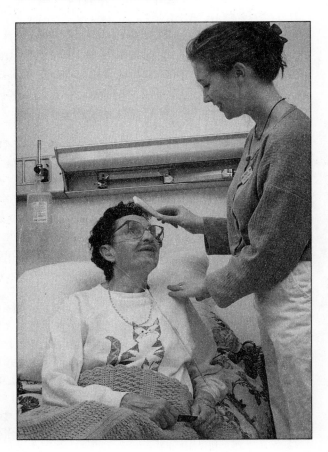

Figure 5–3 Sincere compliments assure clients that they are still worthy of respect.

nursing diagnoses   the specific issues in a client's recovery that are solely the responsibility of the nurse

When the nurse on the case determines the appropriate **nursing diagnoses** (nursing care problems) for that client, they became the basis for the nursing care plan and the HCA care plan. At this time, the nurse also defines the client's long-term and short-term goals for the home health agency's period of care. Client goals must be established to provide the health care team with a communication tool. This includes the HCA who will be expected to have an understanding of the goals and the ability to observe the client's progress in reaching these goals.

The HCA is the health care provider most often in the home communicating with the client and the family. Many times, important information is obtained during one of the HCA's visits. The HCA who specializes in care of the client who has had a stroke will have an increased knowledge and awareness of the problems that could hinder the accomplishment of reaching the client's goals. It is important for the HCA to:

- know the goals
- know the possible problems that hinder recovery
- report these problems or changes to the supervisor so the nurse and physician can decide on a course of action to take

When a long-term goal is defined, there are usually several short-term goals necessary to achieve the long-term one. The following is an example of client goals for a CVA case.

Long-Term Goal
- to achieve optimal level of health and functioning through restoring and/or maintaining motor, sensory, and cognitive function affected by a vascular lesion in the brain

Short-Term Goals

compliance   the acceptance of medical instructions and medications by the client

- verbalize nature of disease process, type of CVA, risk factors, importance of **compliance** with prescribed treatment regimen, signs and symptoms of new or recurring problems to report to home health nurse or physician
- demonstrate compliance with prescribed diet, dietary restrictions, adequate hydration
- demonstrate prescribed measures to assist client with problems related to dysphagia, chewing, and feeding difficulties
- verbalize purpose of nutritional supplements
- weigh weekly/record/report excessive weight loss to physician
- demonstrate compliance with prescribed medication therapy, identify side effects, toxicity
- verbalize importance and demonstrate compliance with prescribed anticoagulant therapy, safety factors with taking, adverse reactions are to be reported to physician, measures to control any bleeding

- verbalize importance of prescribed blood coagulation studies and other diagnostic lab work
- demonstrate compliance with prescribed exercise program and planned rest periods
- identify risk factors for falls and injuries, safety measures with ambulation and daily activities
- demonstrate progressive ambulation and self-care activities with use of unaffected side and use of ambulatory aids and self-help devices
- demonstrate compliance with prescribed measures in care of immobilized client
- verbalize predisposing factors to constipation, specific measures to improve bowel function
- demonstrate compliance with prescribed bowel and bladder program
- demonstrate catheter care and management as prescribed
- demonstrate compliance with speech therapy program for maximized communication skills
- demonstrate compliance with prescribed physical and occupational therapy programs for alterations in functional skills and self-care activities
- demonstrate effective coping mechanisms to adapt to altered body image and changes in lifestyle

The HCA does not need to be concerned with the setting of goals because that is a nursing function. The nursing care plan is created by the nurse and focuses on determining goals for each individual client. The goals vary as much as the clients. However, the HCA does need to be aware of these as a specialist caring for the client who has had a stroke. The HCA is an important part of the team working to achieve these goals in the period of time allowed by Medicare or the insurance company for this client's home health program.

The most important aspect of setting short- and long-term goals is to determine the expected patient outcomes of these goals. Nursing care plans are structured so that the nurse and physician can begin the plan of care by first establishing the outcomes, statements of patient/family/caregiver behaviors that are measured and observed during the process of care. They should have a target date of accomplishment based on the individual client and that client's expected progress.

Once the client's mental state is positive and motivation is being demonstrated, the rehabilitation phase can move toward recovery. This is done by setting client goals and constantly evaluating them until recovery is completed.

The goals which the health care team, the family, and the client set should include short-term goals, such as relearning to brush teeth, to long-range goals, such as dancing again. These goals are different for each client, depending on the individual's disease condition and real abilities to recover those lost skills. However, there are four major goals in the rehabilitation phase common to all clients who have had a stroke:

- retrain for the most mobility
- restore the highest level of ADLs and self-care
- improve thinking ability
- restructure a role in the family and/or community

We will look at each of these goals and discuss what the challenges are for the whole team and for the client.

Mobility

The first goal in the rehabilitation phase is for the client to be retrained for the highest degree of **mobility** possible for that client, taking all influencing factors into consideration. Influencing factors affecting the outcome of the client's mobility will include the following:

- severity and reversible effects of the stroke to the voluntary muscles involved
- age and overall health of the client
- effectiveness of preventative measures in the earlier stages of recovery
- amount of thought process damage, including ability to follow instructions
- degree of family/caregiver involvement and commitment
- motivation level of the client
- emotional state of the client and family
- degree of client's ability to perform any self-care functions
- ability of the health care team to motivate and instruct the client and family

As discussed in Chapter 2, in the early phases of the stroke, correct positioning is crucial in preventing contractures, maintaining good body alignment, preventing skin breakdown, and preventing debilitating nerve damage. Turning and changing the client's position is important until the client is mobile and moving on his or her own.

As the client begins to recover from the brain damage caused by the CVA, treatment rather than prevention of inactivity begins. Retraining for mobility involves the affected extremities by exercising them to increase mobility and strength. The repeating of exercise patterns of motion sends new messages to the brain

mobility   ability to move

over and over again until they become as natural to movement as the old messages prior to the stroke. ROM exercises are frequently ordered, and designed and directed by the PT. Frequent short exercise periods conserve the client's energy better than long strenuous periods. Each muscle strengthens as the exercises are repeated on a regular schedule. The unaffected side may require assistance in movement for a while until strength and motion are restored. The HCA may be asked to provide the necessary passive ROM techniques to assist the client. Eventually, the ROMs will become more of an active program in which the client does the exercises on his or her own without the HCA's help. The focus of exercise at this point in the rehabilitation is on:

- flexibility
- strength
- coordination
- balance
- endurance (not showing signs of physical exhaustion such as shortness of breath, rapid pulse, chest pain, or cyanosis [gray color due to oxygen-poor blood])

The client is never exercised beyond discomfort to a body part. The PT begins to strengthen the client's arm and leg muscles in preparation for walking and ambulating. The client should become confident of strength and balance in a sitting position before walking is attempted. The client who is hemiplegic will have a loss of balance which must be restored in the sitting position. The HCA who first assists the client must proceed slowly and have a good knowledge of proper body mechanics as well as transferring skills so no injuries to the client or the HCA occur. The important special procedures for assisting the hemiplegic client are:

- sitting and balanced
- standing and balanced
- wheelchair practice
- walking practice

The 10 steps of retraining for mobility are:

1. Proper positioning.
2. ROM in bed (Passive, Passive-active, and Active).
3. Self-turning and moving in bed.
4. Sitting/balance (with assistance or without assistance).
5. Sitting transfer; bed to chair.
6. Standing/balance.
7. Standing transfers (with assistance or without assistance).
8. Wheelchair (with assistance or without assistance).

9. Walking (with assistance or without personal assistive devices).
10. Ambulating all day by self.

The following are guidelines for assisting clients to ambulate:

- assess the client's endurance first
- know the client's exercise plan and what the client may and may not do
- if necessary, use two individuals to assist (especially if balance is poor)
- stand on weaker side
- use a transfer belt
- place a cane on the stronger side (Figure 5–4)
- if using assistive devices, use good body mechanics
- always have client in proper walking shoes
- use encouragement and praise; never criticize or show your frustration
- be patient and positive

Not all clients who have had a CVA will progress at the same rate. Setting short-term goals rather than long-term goals is important. For example, emphasize that today the client will move 10 feet more than he or she did yesterday, rather than stating the goal is to walk all the way to the bathroom by tomorrow.

Activities of Daily Living/Self-Care

ADLs are those functions people do everyday to care for themselves including bathing, eating, showering, nail care, hair care, mouth care, dressing, and elimination.

Personal care procedures for clients who have had a stroke are to return the client to caring for himself or herself. It is important

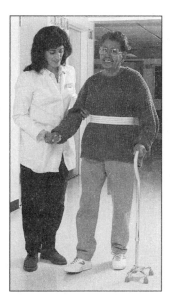

Figure 5–4 The patient holds the cane on her strong side. She puts the cane forward first, then the weak leg, and then the strong leg. The nursing assistant stands on her weak side.

that the client feels that progress is being made during this long rehabilitation period. Oftentimes, providing their own personal care in small stages is the only real progress clients feel is happening. Some of the reasons that clients who have had a stroke cannot perform personal care may be:

- weakness of the arms and shoulders
- inability to remember the sequence of a task
- poor judgment
- inability to remember items and their use for personal care
- depression
- indifference to appearance

Some of the personal care activities that these clients have problems with are:

- bathing
- shaving
- mouth care and denture care
- hair care
- skin care
- nail care
- foot care

When assisting the client with personal care, the HCA must have patience, and explain slowly and carefully what is to be done. The occupational therapist or nurse will set up techniques for the client and caregivers to follow. The following are guidelines for assisting functionally limited persons with personal care:

1. Do not begin to assist the client before he or she is ready, both physically and emotionally.
2. Follow the plan set up by the therapist or the nurse.
3. Provide a safe environment for the client.
4. Assemble and place all equipment where the client can reach it easily.
5. Remind the client of areas he or she may forget.
6. Always wash the involved arm or leg first.
7. Demonstrate the proper technique, such as rinsing and patting dry.
8. Assist the client with controlling the temperature of water.
9. Offer to perform personal care in areas the client cannot reach easily.

The HCA should always use the time with the client to observe his or her body and condition.

Returning the client to self-care is a long-term goal in all home health care situations. This is especially true for clients who have lost the ability to care for themselves to a large degree. The amount of self-care rehabilitation possible depends on the client, and the degree of injury involved. There is a big difference between returning the client with arthritis to self-care and that of a survivor of a brain injury. The main goal, however, is for the health care team to determine the optimal level that can be obtained, and then to strive to meet that level, whatever it might be. Because every human being has the need to feel useful, self-care must include some functions that the client considers useful.

Minimal self-care can simply entail performing ADLs such as feeding and bathing. At the other extreme, self-care might involve helping a client who has had a stroke learn to drive a car again. Many of these clients go home to lead normal lives through the rehabilitation process. Independence is a major factor, and may mean simply performing ADLs or being back in the workplace and collecting a pay check on a regular basis. The health care team must all agree on the plan and the goals and discuss them with the client and the family on an on-going basis.

The return to self-care must involve the client's physical, psychological, socioeconomic, spiritual, and environmental status. The therapist and all the members of the health care team must consider all five areas before a comprehensive self-care plan can be considered successful.

People learn to do ADLs as children. Clients who have had a stroke must relearn these skills. Because of perceptual deficits, a client may not be able to:

- organize an ADL task, such as gather necessary equipment or know what to do first, second, and so forth
- use judgement for appropriate tasks at the correct times, such as putting on clothes before shoes
- recognize ADL tools formerly used, such as a razor to shave
- grasp ADL tools, such as a comb or toothbrush

The client will feel better if he or she is wearing clothes rather than bedclothes as quickly as possible in the rehabilitation phase. Clothing should fit well and be easy to put on and take off. Velcro is a great substitute for zippers and buttons, and can be replaced easily on the client's favorite clothes.

Dressing is easier if the client does as much as possible in a sitting position. Clothing should be placed on the affected side first (see Procedure 17, Dressing the Client, in Chapter 7). A large mirror may help the client to see what he or she is doing. Dressing skills, especially putting on shoes and socks, are difficult skills to relearn for the client who has had a stroke. Even making choices of what to wear may upset the client early in the program. The client should be encouraged to do as much as possible according to his or her limitations.

Thinking

The entire health care team plays a role in assessing and retraining the client who has had a stroke to improve thinking ability. Some of the techniques used are based on visual and verbal clues that reprogram the brain to respond to these clues and process resulting thoughts and actions. A neuropsychologist is a specialist trained to evaluate and treat brain-damaged individuals. The program includes therapy as well as counseling to create new problem-solving abilities for the client. These clients are easily distracted and have memory problems, so this is the slowest of the rehabilitation processes. Patience on the part of the caregivers is essential to success (Figure 5–5).

Family Role

Returning the client to previous roles played before the illness comes late in the rehabilitation phase of recovery. This may require special counseling when the skills to return completely to former roles are not there. This may mean giving up a job or simply giving up the role of decision-maker for the family. There are many losses involved in this area and some clients find this the most difficult loss to handle. A man who was formerly the breadwinner and head of his household who must retire early and watch his wife become the outside worker will probably experience a great loss of self-esteem.

The attitude and acceptance of the family is an important factor in how the client handles such losses. If the family is now expected to care for the client on a 24-hour basis, the stresses are even greater. The medical social worker plays an important part in recommending assistance to the family in the way of home health aides, meal services, day care, respite centers, and stroke support groups. When the family responds negatively to the client, emotions in the home become very tense. The client may feel like a burden or become overly demanding in an attempt to have his or her needs met.

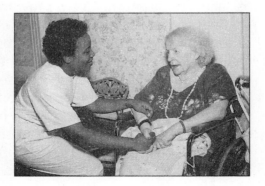

Figure 5–5   Patience is essential during the recovery process.

Three areas the client needs to resolve in restructuring a role in the family and community are:

1. Money, including earning power and expenses of the illness.
2. Household tasks and decisions which may include client care.
3. Access to the outside world, including transportation.

It is important that the client and family be realistic in their expectations of the client's return to former roles. Table 5–1 is a timetable for rehabilitation of the client who has had a stroke.

SUMMARY

This chapter emphasizes the importance of motivation and the setting of short- and long-term goals in the rehabilitation and restorative phase of the client who has had a CVA. The ten steps of retraining for mobility include the roles that HCAs play in assisting clients to walk and ambulate. Returning the client to self-care at whatever level he or she may achieve is the goal each HCA must set with each and every client. After one client has

Table 5–1

Timetable	Phase	Rehabilitation Process
Day 1–3	Acute Phase	• Assess cognitive losses • Position correctly • Assess communication • Maintain nutrition • Dangle extremities if possible
Day 3–5	Early Rehabilitation	• Sit in chair • Bedside commode • Use wheelchair and transfer with assistance • Go to PT • Use splints or sling • Continue to check elimination • Evaluate for and begin OT for ADLs • Observe food and fluid intake
Day 6–10	Rehabilitation Phase	• Bladder training • Assist wheelchair to bed to BR • Learn gait training • Begin ADL practice sessions to self-care • Speech therapy/water swallowing
2–3 Weeks	To Rehabilitation Center	• Prepare for home-outpatient therapy • Assistive devices to improve gait and ambulation • Family sessions and education • Continue bladder training
3–6 Weeks	Home Care	• HCA to assist home maintenance • Provide safe environment • Evaluate progress periodically; return to self-care

reached success, there will always be more clients who need the experience of the HCA to motivate and assist them in reaching their personal goals.

CASE STUDY

The client who is assigned to you is refusing to do anything for herself and demanding that you give her a complete bed bath. Your care plan states she should assist herself with ADLs. What is your plan of action?

REVIEW QUESTIONS

1. To set goals hoping to return to a former state of function is to set _____ goals.
2. _____ _____ is the end result the client and the team are hoping and planning to reach.
3. The need or desire to do something is called _____.
4. ADL is A _____ of D _____ L _____.
5. Which of the following is *not* a major goal common to all clients who have had a stroke?
   a. improve thinking
   b. restore self-care
   c. improve mobility
   d. learn to cook
6. Factors that affect the outcome of the client's mobility include:
   a. motivation
   b. age
   c. health
   d. all of the above
7. The health care person most often in the home with the client is the:
   a. therapist
   b. HCA
   c. nurse
   d. physician

8. Compliance by the client is demonstrated by:
   a. taking medications correctly
   b. demonstrating self-care activities as taught
   c. sleeping at night
   d. a and b only

9. True or False? The client should have a positive mental state and demonstrate motivation before the rehabilitation phase begins.

10. True or False? Nurses and physicians establish expected outcomes.

11. True or False? Relearning to brush teeth is an example of a long-term goal.

12. True or False? Mobility is usually not a factor with a client who has had a stroke.

13. Unscramble the following key term from the chapter: cmpnaiolec _____

CHAPTER 6

Home Care Aide Roles and Functions

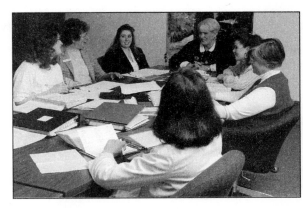

OBJECTIVES

Upon reading this chapter and completing the review questions, the home care aide should be able to:

1. List the aspects and importance of communication, cooperation, and coordination.
2. Describe the general rules basic to all documentation.
3. State the additional areas of concern for clients who have had a stroke.
4. Describe case conferences, case managers, medical plans of treatment, and the role of the HCA.

KEY TERMS

case conferences
case manager
cooperation
coordination

documentation
HCA care plan
signs
symptoms

INTRODUCTION

cooperation common effort

coordination smooth interaction by all members of the team toward a common goal

As the HCA is given more responsibility through specialization, the nurse and the HCA will become a closely working team. The three Cs, the important aspects involved in this team, are communication, **cooperation**, and **coordination**.

The HCAs' roles and functions will be increasing and become more specific to caring for the client with unique needs, such as one who has had a stroke. Some of the new roles and functions for HCAs caring for the client are:

1. Providing personal care to the client who has had a stroke by assisting with bathing and dressing, but encouraging the

client to do as much as possible to return to the highest level of self-care.

2. Providing management of the home to make it a clean and safe environment in which the client can recuperate.

3. Using principles of good body mechanics to conserve energy and prevent injury to both the HCA and the client.

4. Understanding the principles of rehabilitation to reinforce PT, OT, and ST programs.

5. Using proper transfer and ambulation techniques to safely increase mobility and strength in the client.

6. Providing psychosocial support to the client and/or family.

7. Understanding the skilled nurse's role and observing and reporting to the supervisor all changes in the client's progress.

8. Participating in case conferences.

9. Offering procedures, such as range of motion exercises and positioning, to assist the client in recuperation.

OBSERVATION AND REPORTING

The HCA's roles and functions in caring for clients who have had a stroke center around proper communication and the use of communication tools. This includes observing and reporting the client's condition as well as properly documenting the client's care, changes, and status. The HCA care plan and visit notes are useful communication tools which the specially trained HCA should use consistently and properly.

The HCA will spend more time with the client than the other members of the health care team. Therefore, other members of the health care team will rely on the HCA to observe the client carefully and report changes and problems to the supervisor so they are kept constantly informed. Figure 6–1 shows the communication process between the client, HCA, and other members of the health care team. The **case manager** is the nurse who coor-

case manager   coordinator; person in charge of the care of a specific client

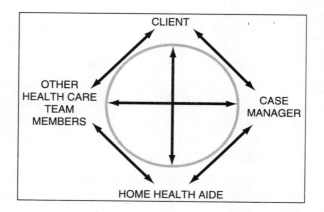

Figure 6–1 The HCA interacts with all members of the health care team.

dinates all the care the client is receiving. The supervisor and case manager may not be the same person, but they will keep each other informed on a day-to-day basis.

Some questions the HCA might ask the client to obtain more information before reporting to the supervisor include the following:

1. What is the problem? (pain, weakness)

2. Where is the problem? The client should point to where the problem is exactly.

3. When has the client had this problem before?

4. Is there any treatment that has been done that makes it worse or better? (heat, ice, Tylenol®)

Some specific basic observations of clients who have had a stroke are:

- changes in skin status (breakdown, reddened areas, bruises, sores, bleeding, cuts)
- changes in walking (limping, weakness, unsteadiness, paralysis, shuffle)
- pain with movement
- swelling of limbs and joints
- deformity or permanent misshaping of a body part
- hot or cold extremity
- functional loss
- shaking, twitching, and numbness of arms or legs
- changes in eye status (sensitivity to light, double vision, fixed pupils)
- complaints of headache, or an observable change in mental status (slow to respond, confused, anxious, excessive fatigue)
- changes in elimination (bladder or bowel incontinence, or painful urination or defecation)
- family or caregiver stress that could affect the client's recovery
- changes in the client's interest and motivation in returning to self-care
- any equipment not working properly

DOCUMENTATION

documentation the written account of care given

Documentation is the written account of all activities, procedures done, and observations made when health caregivers are in the client's home. The client's record or chart contains documentation from all members of the care team including the nurse, physician, therapist, and the HCA. The daily visit form has space for documentation for each and every treatment, procedure, and observation. The client's record is a legal document;

therefore, careful and accurate recording is very important. The following are general guidelines for documentation:

1. The client record is written evidence of the care given, the client's response, and the outcome of the care.

2. The client's record reflects changes in orders and in the client's condition so all members of the health care team can keep current.

3. The client's record is a communication tool on which the plan for care is evaluated and updated.

4. The client's record is a written document required by insurance companies and regulatory agencies to validate the care given.

5. The client's record may be used in a court to prove that care was given and observations documented.

6. The client's record in home care is the basis for reimbursement or payment for care provided.

Every agency has its own type of records and forms. The specially trained HCA should receive a complete orientation as to the type of paperwork used in the agency and become familiar with the documentation policies of the employer. Some of the forms the HCA might use are:

- ADL sheets (Figure 6–2)
- daily visit forms
- graph sheets for TPRs
- HCA care plan
- client information sheet

COOPERATION

Helpful Hint: The nurse has been called the "heart of home care" and the HCA the "heartbeat" by the National Association of Home Care.

The HCA spends more time with the client than any other member of the health care team and should be the one to observe the client for changes in condition, especially if the changes are negative. The HCA is the eyes and ears of the nurse and it is his or her responsibility to observe, document, and report everything the nurse needs to know to manage the case. The HCA uses cooperation (willingness to act jointly with others) to interact and participate with others in the client's care.

signs client changes that can be seen, felt, heard or smelt

symptoms client's stated complaints

The HCA reports **signs** which are changes seen, heard, felt, or smelt and **symptoms**, those complaints the clients describe. Who should the HCA report these signs and symptoms to? The answer is the supervisor. When the HCA reports to the supervisor, he or she must *also* document the same information in written form on the client's record.

Name Cedrone, Paul									Room 311

Activities of Daily Living

DATE	7/14								
I. DIET:	7-3	3-11	11-7	7-3	3-11	11-7	7-3	3-11	11-7
A. MEALS-AMT. EATEN	all all								
B. NOURISHMENTS									
II. PERSONAL HYGIENE									
A. Complete bath									
B. Assist									
C. Self	√								
D. Shower/tub bath									
E. Mouth care	X2								
F. Peri care									
G. Back care									
III. ACTIVITY									
A. Bed rest	√								
B. Dangle									
C. C&B									
DBRP									
E. Ambulate									
F. ROM									
IV. Elimination									
A. Bowels	X1								
1. Amount	small								
2. Consistency	liq.								
3. Enema and results									
4. Incontinent									
B. Bladder									
1. Voided	X3								
2. Catheterized									
3. Catheter care									
4. Incontinent									
V. TREATMENTS									
1. Leg exercised TCDB									
2. Antiembol. stockings - removed and replaced									
3. Dressing changes									
4. Irrigations									
5. Soaks - hot packs, cold packs									
VI. SPECIMENS (Specify)									
VII. DIAGNOSTIC TESTS									
VIII. OTHER	stool gu neg								
IX. SIDE RAILS UP	↑↓								
X. SLEEP (naps, well, poorly)	naps								
XI. Signature	S. Lopez NA								

Figure 6–2 Example of an ADL form for documenting client behaviors

There are some general rules that are basic to all documentation. They include the following:

1. Recording should be descriptive and a note written about each complaint or problem.

2. Using words that are descriptive rather than general terms, such as "normal" or "good."

3. Writing should be neat.

4. Recording should be done in black ink.

5. Recording should begin with the date and time and end with a signature and title.

6. Recording should have the time a change was noticed and in long-term cases, a note at least every two hours.

7. When quoting client symptoms, use quotation marks.

8. All attempts to report to the supervisor should be carefully documented. If a message is left, a note should be written on the record describing who was spoken to, the date, and the time.

9. Errors should not be erased, but a line drawn through the wrong entry, "error" written next to it, and the HCA's initials.

10. Abbreviations should only be those accepted by the HCA's agency.

11. The HCA should only chart his or her own observations and activities, not those of another HCA. The HCA's signature legally states that he or she did the procedure and documented it.

12. If a new page is added, the client's name must be on each new page, as well as the time, date, and signature written again.

The following is an example of documentation for a problem occurring in a client who has had a stroke.

The HCA arrives at Mrs. Edna Cromwell's home at 8 AM to find that she is still in bed, even though yesterday she had gotten up unassisted to the bedside commode. The client is six weeks post-CVA and has been progressing well both in activity and in strength. She tells you, "I got up during the night to go to the bathroom on the commode chair, and lost my balance. I slipped, but didn't fall on the floor. I did hurt myself."

The HCA should:

- take vital signs
- observe the client's body
- report the complaints to the supervisor immediately

The HCA's documentation should reflect the following:

> 8:00 AM—On arrival, found Mrs. Edna Cromwell lying in bed with an expression of pain, and crying. Client states, "I got up during the night to go to the bathroom on the commode chair, and lost my balance. I slipped, but didn't fall on the floor. I did hurt myself." B/P—140/90; TPR—98.2—90—24. Supervisor notified of client's condition.
>
> 8:15 AM—Bath given to client in bed. Supervisor awaiting response from physician and skilled nurse due at this home when orders received.
>
> 9:00 AM—Nurse arrived with new orders. Care plan updated. Cold compresses applied to left hip. No bruises, swelling, or redness noted at this time.
>
> 10:00 AM—Client states, "Pain is gone and I feel much better."

Helpful Hint: Your notes should reflect your level of professionalism as well as your attitude. Write carefully and accurately.

Helpful Hint: The agency is paid by the insurance company for the visit. Your client and your own signature are legal proof that the visit was indeed completed.

HOME CARE AIDE CARE PLAN AND DAILY VISIT FORM

HCA care plan plan the HCA follows which is created by the nurse and updated every two weeks

The contents of the **HCA care plan** for the client who has had a stroke is determined by the nurse on the case based on the condition of the patient and the physician's orders. An example of a care plan appropriate for all types of clients is shown in Figure 6–3. The "specific treatment and instructions" section may be adapted by the nurse for the client who has had a stroke. The nurse can make the HCA care plan individualized for each client based on specific nursing diagnoses, the client's activities of daily living, that client's goals, and expected outcomes. As the client's condition improves or changes, the nurse continually updates the care plan in the "changes" section. The HCA care plan shown

RIVERVIEW HOME HEALTH SERVICE
8987 Walkman Ave
Parkhurst, Nebraska
Client Care Plan / Progress Notes

WT. 146 TEMP. 98 BP 114/80 P 70 R 14 MD CONTACT C. Boylston
HOMEBOUND DUE TO Spinal Cord Injury - Paraplegia MEN. STATUS Alert - Coherent

PROBLEMS	INTERVENTIONS	TIME	PLAN	OUTCOME
① Potential altered	maintain high-calorie, low-residue, high-protein diet		Morning Care	Tol. well
nutrition: less than	Reduce high calcium and gas-producing foods	0700	Breakfast	ate entire meal
body requirements	Provide balanced meals	0815	Commode	soft formed stool
	morning and evening	0900	Bath, Cath Care,	
	supplements	0945	ROM	
			up in wheelchair	Tolerated well
② Potential for disuse	exercise to tolerance avoid fatigue. ROM	1030	6 ʒ High Cal drink	
syndrome related to	Turn and reposition q 1 hr.	1045	Returned to Bed	
effects of immobility	up in wheelchair B.I.D. encourage self-care	1130	Positioned on Rt side	
	activities to tolerance		Positioned on Back	
③ alteration in bowel	Stool Softener, Glycerine	1230	Lunch	½ tuna sand/Tea
elimination: constipation	Suppositories, enemas, PRN.			
	Check for BM q 3 days		up in wheelchair	
		1330	Returned to Bed	
④ Potential for infection	Routine catheter care	1430	Positioned on left side.	
related to indwelling	Change per routine schedule		Watching T.V.	
Foley catheter		1500		
⑤ Self-concept disturbance	encourage verbalization of feelings and fears			
related to effects of	encourage independence. Be positive and reassuring			
limitations				

DAILY SUMMARY
Diet and supplements taken fairly well. Activity tolerated. Muscles soft but some tone. Soft formed stool. Expressed frustration during transfers from bed to wheelchair. Enjoys reading and watching T.V. Seems to be gaining some confidence in transfer activities

Visit Date ______ Pt. Last Name, First Initial Mitchell, D. Employee Signature Ruthy Chek, CNA
Nursing Supervisor Report

Joint Visit in Home ______
Conference ______
Patient's personal care and comfort measures by home aide are: superior ___; good ___; satisfactory ___; need improvement ___;
Services provided were appropriate ___; inappropriate ___.

Comments

Figure 6–3 Sample client care plan

in Figure 6–4 is divided into nine main sections to be included on each visit. These are:

1. extremities
2. skin
3. nutrition
4. home maintenance
5. exercise/activity level
6. ambulation
7. personal care
8. elimination
9. mental status

For the client who has had a stroke, in addition to these routine areas of concern, the nurse would most likely emphasize:

- skin care
- prevention of deformities
- reinforcement of the client's exercise program
- gait training
- safety precautions
- bowel and bladder retraining
- observation of changes in rehabilitation status
- reinforcement of speech program
- safe ambulation and transfers
- any measure to reestablish self-care

In order to accommodate the increased HCA activities and documentation, it will be necessary for the care plan to be specific to the client. A daily visit form has been developed to guide the HCA in what procedures are to be done at each visit. There are observation requirements for each visit. There are also specific procedures for care that are to be performed on some clients and not on others. Therefore, the care plan is divided into routine tasks that should be done on every visit and those which the nurse will instruct the HCA to do for that specific client on that visit. The HCA care plan and daily visit form are important communication tools, and it is important that the HCA make them a part of his or her routine documentation.

COORDINATION

Coordination of the team means they work together in a harmonious manner interacting equally, toward common goals, and with a coordinator or leader who keeps each person focused and informed. The home care manager is usually the coordinator for each client case. This person or the agency may have a nurse

Helpful Hint: Never hesitate to ask the nurse or your supervisor a question about the client. They want you to keep informed.

Name _____		No: _____		Diagnosis: _____	
Home Care Aide: _____				Date of visit: _____	
Date of Discharge: _____		Nurse: _____			

Routine Care:		Date:	Documentation:	Sign:
I.	Observe Extremities			
	A. Temperature			
	B. Color			
	C. Numbness			
	D. Pain			
	E. Ulcerations			
	F. Tingling			
II.	Observe Skin			
	A. Reddened areas			
	B. Positioning for pressure points			
	C. Ulcerations/blisters			
	D. Wound			
III.	Observe/assist Nutrition			
	A. Adequate fluid intake and output			
	B. Fiber diet for bowel training			
	C. Encourage/restriction fluids for bladder training			
	D. Special diet			
IV.	Observe/assist Home Maintainance			
	A. Patient totally dependent			
	B. Patient needs some assistance			
	C. Patient independent (10–100%) _____			
	D. Self-care			
V.	Observe/assist Exercise/Activity Level			
	A. PT exercise as ordered			
	B. OT or ST exercise as ordered			
	C. ROM exercises			
	1. Passive			
	2. Active			
	3. Assistive			
	D. Patient diability level (10–100%) _____			
VI.	Observe/assist Ambulation			
	A. Safety precautions			
	B. Visual problems			
	C. Unsteady gait			
	D. Assisting devices			
	E. Environment			
VII.	Observe/assist Personal Care			
	A. Bathing			
	B. Oral care			
	C. Hair care			
	D. Shaving			
	E. Nail care			
VIII.	Observe/assist Elimination			
	A. Incontinent			
	B. Constipation			
	C. Diarrhea			
	D. Frequency/burning on urination			
	E. Adequate/inadequate fluid intake			
IX.	Observe Mental Status			
	A. Depression			
	B. Confusion			
	C. Forgetfulness			
	D. State of agitation			
	E. Stress			
	F. Oriented			
	G. Impulsiveness			
	H. Activity			

Specific Treatments/Procedures:	Date:	Documentation:	Sign:
Skin Care			
Positionioning/Repositioning			
Bowel and Bladder Training			
Gait Training			
Assistive Devices Training			
Return to Self-care Training			
Reinforcement of prescribed Exercise Regimen			
ROM Exercises			
Reinforcement of Speech Exercises			
Logging of Intake and Output			

Figure 6–4 HCA Visit Form for Rehabilitation (Courtesy of Health Education, Inc.)

based in the office to act as coordinator or case manager. This nurse, a PT, or an OT acts as a central information center to which all members of the team report, including the client and family. This may be done by telephone, person-to-person conferences, or case conferences. Many agencies require the field persons on the case, including HCAs, to call in every day so all information is up to date. The case manager cannot make nursing decisions without the proper input from the HCAs, field nurses, and therapists. The physician is included in the coordinator's team and must be called to report changes, problems, lab findings, and for orders required to give proper medical care.

The client's medical plan of treatment is the entire medical plan that the physician orders for the duration of the home health agency's period of caregiving. It includes all the services and treatments to be offered, diet, medications, client goals, expected outcomes, safety concerns, and how often the therapists, nurses, and HCAs visit the client.

CASE CONFERENCES

case conferences meetings of all members of the health care team to analyze the client's case

Case conferences are meetings held periodically with all members of the health care team to analyze the management of the client's case and to point out problem areas and possible changes in the care plan. Figure 6–5 shows the members of the healthcare team meeting for a case conference. In CVA cases, case conferences should be held every 2 to 4 weeks. It is important that all the disciplines involved in the case have input and that documentation be accurate on a case conference form. The

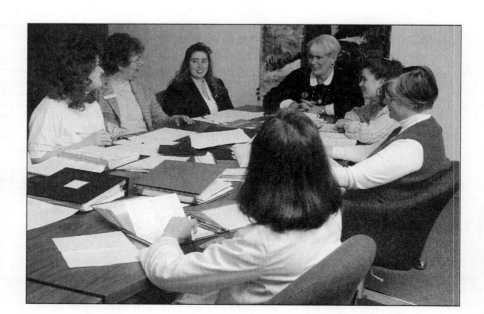

Figure 6–5 Case conferences are attended by the members of the interdisciplinary team.

HCA on the case should be included in the conference and the HCA care plan updated at this time.

The specially trained HCA who participates in case conferences provides important information to the other members of the team. The members involved in case conferencing may include the physician, the physical therapist, the occupational therapist, the speech therapist, the dietitian, the medical social worker, the skilled nurse, and the home care aide. Sometimes case conferencing is done over the telephone with case conference calls. It is the responsibility of all health care workers to keep up to date on the results of case conferences. If the HCA misses the conference, it is still his or her responsibility to obtain the updated information from the nurse or supervisor.

The case conference includes the following important areas:

- common team goals
- team members' care plans and treatment plans
- problems and problem-solving
- client status through an evaluation process
- new orders to the care plan
- client goals and outcomes and the progress made toward them

All case conferences should be documented in terms of measurable outcomes for the client. Usually, the skilled nurse is the case manager and, therefore, responsible for the documentation and the communication to other members of the team. The HCA should prepare for case conferences carefully and professionally as an important member of the management team.

As the team prepares the client for discharge, it becomes more and more important that case conferences be held and goals assessed.

> **Helpful Hint:** There are times when the HCA's input will make a great difference as to the success of the case conference.

SUMMARY

The three Cs, communication, cooperation, and coordination, are key to the HCA's roles and functions in caring for clients who have had a CVA. The basic skills of observation, reporting, and documentation become even more important when the HCA is a member of a team which needs to be kept constantly informed. These skills grow more valuable and sharper with every CVA case in which the HCA is involved. The most valuable HCA is one the nurse is confident will follow the HCA care plan and participate on a professional level in the assignments as ordered by the physician.

CASE STUDY

Your client has refused to cooperate with all members of the team including the three therapists. The case manager has called a case conference to which you have been invited. Should you attend? Why?

REVIEW QUESTIONS

1. The _____ _____ is the basis for the Nursing Care Plan and HCA Care Plan.

2. The _____ is the health care person who communicates most frequently with the client.

3. Two important aspects involved when the HCA and the nurse act as a team are _____ and _____ .

4. Which of the following is *not* included in the HCA Care Plan?

   a. nutrition

   b. activity

   c. PT goals

   d. personal care

5. Choose the area or areas of concern that should be emphasized in caring for clients who have had a stroke.

   a. self-care

   b. skin care

   c. safety

   d. all of the above

6. True or False? All clients who require rehabilitation need bowel and bladder training.

7. True or False? Clients should be encouraged to do as much for themselves as possible and allowed to do so, even if it takes more time.

8. True or False? Some clients may not remember their progress from one day to the next.

9. True or False? The client's goals and expected outcomes must be considered on a 24-hour basis to obtain the best results.

10. True or False? The physician writes the treatment plan.

11. True or False? The HCA writes the HCA Care Plan.

12. Unscramble the following key term from this chapter: pmsymsto _____

CHAPTER 7

Client Care Procedures

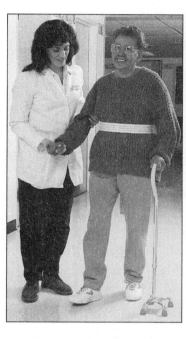

OBJECTIVES

Upon reading this chapter and completing the review questions, the home care aide should be able to:

1. List the challenges the HCA and the client who has had a CVA must meet to return to self-care.

2. Define ambulation and gait training.

3. Describe elimination, nutrition, and home environment in client care.

4. Demonstrate the following:
   - Procedure 1 Assisting the Client to Walk with Crutches, Walker, or Cane
   - Procedure 2 Caring for a Urinary Catheter
   - Procedure 3 Connecting the Leg Bag
   - Procedure 4 Emptying a Drainage Unit
   - Procedure 5 Training and Retraining Bowels
   - Procedure 6 Insertion of a Rectal Suppository
   - Procedure 7 Administering a Commercial Enema
   - Procedure 8 Retraining the Bladder
   - Procedure 9 Measuring and Recording Fluid Intake and Output

- Procedure 10 Assisting the Client who can Feed Self
- Procedure 11 Feeding the Dependent Client
- Procedure 12 Positioning the Client in Supine Position
- Procedure 13 Positioning the Client in Lateral Side-Laying Position
- Procedure 14 Positioning the Client in Prone Position
- Procedure 15 Positioning the Client in Fowler's Position
- Procedure 16 Special Skin Care and Pressure Sores
- Procedure 17 Dressing and Undressing the Client
- Procedure 18 Performing Passive Range of Motion (ROM) Exercises

KEY TERMS

bowel and bladder retraining

functional limitation

gait training

home maintenance

pressure ulcers

pureed diet

therapeutic (treatment) diets

INTRODUCTION

Caring for clients who have had a CVA can be challenging, even for the specially trained HCA. If the HCA care plan focuses on the following important areas, the care will be comprehensive:

- return to self care
- ambulation and gait training
- elimination, catheter care, and bowel and bladder training
- nutrition/input and output
- home environment
- special procedures including:
  — positioning/transfers
  — skin care
  — assisting dressing
  — ROM

RETURN TO SELF-CARE

The HCA plays an important part in assisting the client to return to self-care. It is the goal for the client from the very first days of the acute phase of the stroke. Knowing how much or how little to do for the client is a judgement every HCA must make, with the rest of the team, for every individual case. If the client will never be able to perform his or her own care, it would be upsetting and frustrating if the team members insist on it. The therapists, nurses, and physician will have a good idea of how much self-care the client will return to by the time the restorative phase is half through. At this point, all professionals will have evaluated the client's functional abilities. The specially trained HCA should keep informed on such evaluations and go to the HCA care plan for changes in Activities of Daily Living status and self-care goals. All of the discussions in the previous chapters now come together to determine the client's self-care abilities and status. All of the five major losses have been evaluated and considered. The complications noted should have been prevented and/or treated, and the seven goals for health care considered before a self-care program is completed.

Self-care for the client who has had a stroke is an ongoing process which peaks during the chronic phase of the stroke (which will be discussed in Chapter 8). However, the process toward self-care is a long and continuous one for these clients. The actual highest possible level of self-care may not be at the level the client hoped for. Disappointment will have to be dealt with and encouragement take its place or there is a risk that the client will begin to regress if he or she does not keep focused and motivated.

AMBULATION AND GAIT TRAINING

Restoring ambulation is usually under the supervision of the PT. However, the HCA cares for the client from day to day and is a factor in the ambulation process. Ambulation means walking. This begins early in the rehabilitation phase when the HCA first assists the client to stand by the bed or chair. Ambulation probably depended on the use of assistive devices early on in the program, but the client may have to use them for life. If the client's body strength and muscle tone have been enhanced with the use of ROM and other PT techniques, when the time comes for walking, the client will have the strength necessary. And if other preventative measures were successful, the client will not have deformities or contractures to interfere with ambulation. The PT is instrumental in teaching the client the proper gait, or walking, technique to use.

gait training   teaching the client the proper gait (walk) with assistive devices

Gait Training (teaching the client to walk) must be ordered by the physician and planned by the physical therapist. However, the HCA is often involved in reinforcement and practice of gait training. Assistive devices involved in gait training include crutches, canes, and walkers which come in many shapes and sizes as we discussed earlier under rehabilitation equipment. Gait training is a rehabilitative exercise to assist the client in improving ambulation. The PT teaches the client to walk correctly on different types of surfaces and how to safely get up from, and down into, a chair.

Safety is an important feature, and the HCA should have plenty of help, particularly if the client is very weak. The area in which the client will be walking must be cleared of clutter and scatter rugs, and there should be no wet areas on the floor. Assistive devices should have safety features such as proper fitting, nonskid tips, and be adaptive to the client's extremity weaknesses. A gait belt should be used for those clients who have a high risk of falling. Figure 7–1A shows how to properly put on a gait belt and Figure 7–1B shows how to use it. The HCA who helps the client ambulate after gait training has been taught should keep in mind the particular limitations of that client. For example, a walker is usually a good choice for clients with generalized weakness in both legs or if one leg is strong enough to bear the client's weight. When ambulating with a cane, the HCA should remember it is used more for balance than for support, and should always be held by the hand on the strong side. If crutches are used for ambulation, the strength of both arms and legs must be considered. If the client has weakness in both legs, forearm crutches work best to provide weight-bearing on the forearms. HCAs should learn how these special crutches are assembled and attached to assist the client when necessary.

Figures 7–2 and 7–3 show how the HCA should support the client when gait training.

There are five basic gaits, and the method used depends on the client's individual problems and limitations:

1. Four-point alternating gait (when the client can bear weight on both feet).

2. Three-point gait (when the client can bear weight on one foot and the affected leg does not touch the ground).

3. Two-point gait (when the client can bear weight on both feet).

4. Swing-to-crutch gait (when the client can bear some weight on both feet but uses the upper arm muscles as strength).

5. Swing-through-crutch gait (requires strong upper arms to lift and swing the body through).

> **Helpful Hint:** Finding help in the home may be a problem. However, don't hesitate to ask the family to assist you to avoid falls or injuries. When in doubt, do not put yourself or the client at risk.

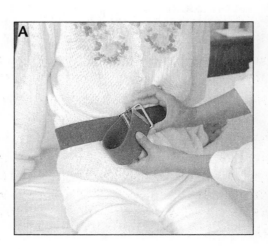 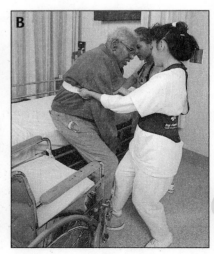

Figure 7–1 (A) A belt is put on the client's waist by first slipping the end through the opening with the teeth. Insert two fingers between the belt and the client's waist to ensure that the belt is not too tight. (B) A transfer belt is used to hold onto the client during transfer.

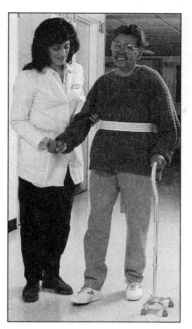

Figure 7–2 Many clients need assistance with walking to prevent them from falling.

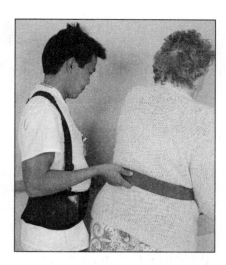

Figure 7–3 This transfer belt is used to hold onto the client while she is ambulating.

A cane is used when there is weakness on one side of the body to help with balance and to support the client. There are one-, three-, and four-pointed canes. The single-tip cane is held on the strong side (if the left leg is weak, the cane is held in the right hand).

A walker is a four-point walking aid which gives the client the most support. The walker is picked up and moved in front of the client and can have wheels or not. Refer to Procedure 1 for assisting the client to walk with a walker, crutches, or a cane.

CLIENT CARE PROCEDURE

1 Assisting the Client to Walk with Crutches, Walker, or Cane

PURPOSE

- To provide support and maintain balance as the client walks.

NOTE: There are three basic walking patterns. With a nonweight-bearing pattern, all the weight is placed on the arms and uninvolved leg. Partial weight-bearing means that minimal weight is placed on the toes. However, most weight is still on the arms and the uninvolved leg.

To walk in a nonweight-bearing pattern, the client uses crutches (see Figure 7–4). The physical therapist measures the client to select the correct length of crutches. The therapist also teaches the client how to walk with them.

To walk in a partial weight-bearing pattern, the client can use crutches but often uses a walker instead. The walker is a curved metal frame with four legs. It is a walking aid that gives maximum stability as the client moves. The client steps forward while holding onto the walker with both hands. Some walkers have wheels so that the client does not have to lift up the walker between steps (see Figure 7–5).

CLIENT CARE PROCEDURE, *continued*

1   Assisting the Client to Walk with Crutches, Walker, or Cane

A cane is used when the client is strong enough to bear full weight on both legs. A standard cane should not be used as a weight-bearing aid. A special cane with four short legs, called a quad cane, is designed to bear a small amount of weight only (see Figure 7–6). A cane is primarily used for balance. Check rubber tips on canes, walkers, and crutches as they wear out quickly if used on sidewalks.

Always have the client wear good supportive shoes with nonskid soles. Instruct clients to pick up their feet and not to look at them but straight ahead.

PROCEDURE

1. Wash your hands. Apply transfer belt unless instructed not to.
2. Always walk on the client's weak side.
3. Walk slightly behind the client holding onto the transfer belt from behind.
4. For the client using crutches, hold onto the transfer belt if the client feels uncomfortable using the crutches (see Figure 7–7A and B).
5. For the client using a walker, instruct the client to place the walker firmly before walking. If the client is strong enough, the walker and the weaker leg can be moved forward at the same time.
6. For the client using a cane (see Figure 7–8A and B), instruct him or her to hold the cane in the hand opposite the weaker leg. For example, if the right ankle has been injured, the client should hold the cane in the left hand.

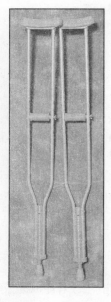

Figure 7–4   Crutches

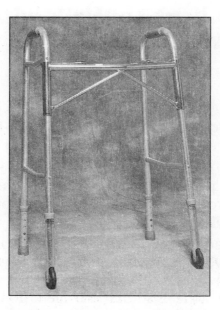

Figure 7–5   Walker with small wheels

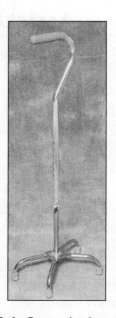

Figure 7–6   Four-point (quad) cane

1   Assisting the Client to Walk with Crutches, Walker, or Cane

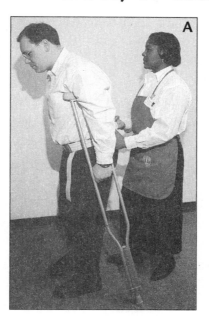 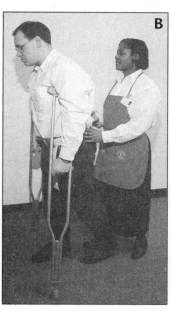

Figure 7–7   Walking with crutches

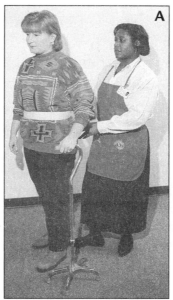 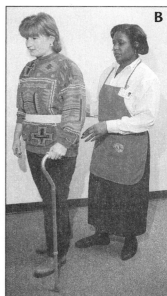

Figure 7–8   Use of various types of canes

7. Balance is a judgmental situation. If the client has poor balance, the aide should support the weak side. If the client has good balance and can walk without assistive devices, the aide should use a transfer belt for safety reasons.

8. Wash your hands at completion of the procedure.

9. Document how far the client walked and his or her reaction.

ELIMINATION, CATHETER CARE, AND BOWEL AND BLADDER TRAINING

The client who has had a stroke will have elimination problems from the beginning. During the acute phase, an indwelling catheter may be inserted into the bladder. The risk of infection is high in clients with catheters in place. To prevent infection, the following measures are important:

1. Make sure that urine is flowing freely through the catheter and that there are no kinks in the tubing.
2. Keep the bag below the level of the bladder to prevent backflow. Attach the bag to the bed frame when the client is in bed.
3. Attach the tubing to the bottom sheet to allow free flow.
4. Secure the catheter to the client's thigh to reduce friction in the urethra.
5. Catheter care (perineal care) should be done every day.
6. The collection bag should be emptied as directed and the urine measured.
7. Report any complaints of pain, burning, or irritation to the supervisor. Chart the color and odor of the urine.
8. Report to the nurse or supervisor if urine is leaking around the catheter.
9. Keep the catheter clean from feces and vaginal drainage.
10. Use a catheter plug or an alcohol soaked 4 x 4 pad if the catheter is separated from the drainage tubing.
11. Always keep bag with the client unless a leg bag is applied.
12. Follow good medical asepsis at all times.
13. Always wash hands before and after handling any urinary equipment.
14. Always wear personal protective equipment.

Refer to Procedure 2 in caring for a urinary catheter, Procedure 3 for connecting the leg bag, and Procedure 4 for emptying a drainage unit. As with all procedures given in this chapter, the HCA should check with the policies and procedures of his or her agency or facility for guidance.

CLIENT CARE PROCEDURE

2   Caring for a Urinary Catheter

PURPOSE

- To clean the area around where the catheter enters the body.
- To prevent infection of the urinary tract.

2   Caring for a Urinary Catheter

- To decrease odors and make the client comfortable.
- To maintain the closed drainage system correctly.

NOTE: The collection bag, tubing, and catheter are referred to as the *closed drainage system* (Figure 7–9). The system should never be disconnected except to reconnect it to a leg bag. The reason the system should not be disconnected is to prevent germs from entering the system (Figure 7–10). Never raise the collection bag higher than the client's bladder. Always check to see if the tubing is lying in the correct position and is not kinked. Never pull on a catheter. If possible, cover bag with a cloth to prevent embarrassment to your client.

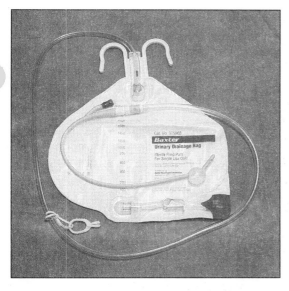

Figure 7–9   Closed drainage system. Note tubing, urine collection bag, and indwelling catheter with bulb inflated.

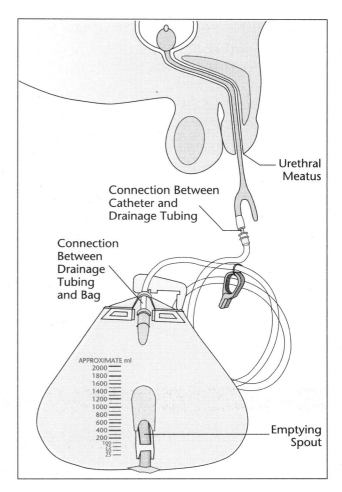

Figure 7–10   Special care must be taken to protect the possible sites of contamination in the closed urinary drainage system.

2   Caring for a Urinary Catheter

PROCEDURE

1. Assemble supplies:
   - disposable gloves
   - antiseptic wipes
   - basin of warm water
   - plastic bag for waste
   - cotton-tipped applicators

2. Wash your hands and apply gloves.

3. Tell client what you plan to do.

4. Position client on his or her back. Expose only the small area where the catheter enters the body. Using soap and warm water or antiseptic wipes, wash area surrounding the catheter. Observe for any skin breakdown, signs of infection, crusting, leakage, or bleeding, which should be reported to the nurse immediately.

5. Using antiseptic wipes or gauze pads dipped in warm water, wipe the catheter tube. make only one stroke with each swab or pad. Discard each wipe after one stroke. Start at the urinary opening and wipe *away* from it. Be careful not to dislodge the catheter. Clean the catheter down to the connection of the drainage tubing.

6. Remove gloves and discard into plastic bag.

7. Check to be sure tubing is coiled on bed (Figure 7–11) and hanging straight down into the drainage container. Check level of urine in the collection bag. Tubing should not be below the collection bag (Figure 7–12). Do not raise collection bag above the level of the client's bladder.

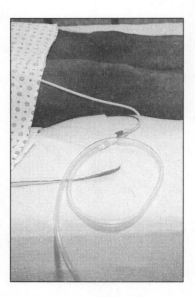

Figure 7-11   Tubing should be placed on top of the leg. The excess tubing should be coiled on the bed.

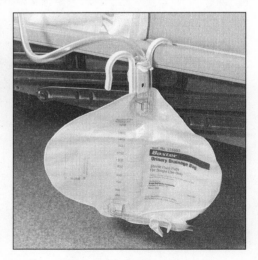

Figure 7-12   The urinary collection bag should be attached to the bed frame. Check to see that the tubing does not fall below the level of the collection bag. Never attach the bag onto the side rails because raising and lowering the rails can dislodge the catheter.

2   Caring for a Urinary Catheter

8. Cover client and discard wastes properly.
9. Wash hands.
10. Document procedure and time, your observations, and client's reaction. Observe color, consistency, and odor of urine, and document.

3   Connecting the Leg Bag

PURPOSE

- To connect a leg urinary collection bag

PROCEDURE

1. Assemble needed equipment:
   - disposable gloves
   - leg bag
   - alcohol wipes
   - paper towels
2. Wash your hands and apply gloves.
3. Tell client what you plan to do.
4. Place paper towel underneath catheter connection area.
5. Use alcohol to disinfect area to be disconnected.
6. Disconnect catheter from tubing. Wipe end of catheter with alcohol (Figure 7–13). Remove cap from end of leg bag and connect leg bag to catheter. Wipe end of bedside drainage bag tubing with alcohol wipe. Place cap on end of closed drainage system.

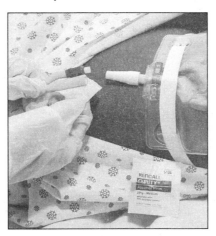

Figure 7–13 Wipe end of catheter with alcohol before connecting leg bag.

3   Connecting the Leg Bag

7. Attach leg straps and bag to client's leg (Figure 7–14). Check to see if the part marked "top of bag" is in the correct position.

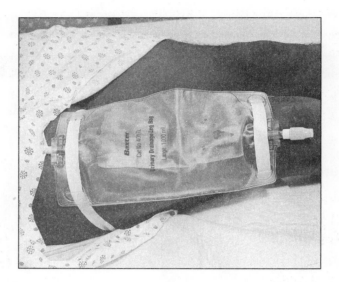

Figure 7–14 Apply leg bag to client's upper leg. Be sure the straps are smooth and not too tight.

8. Empty and measure urine from bedside collection bag.
9. Remove gloves and wash hands.
10. Document procedure completed.

4   Emptying a Drainage Unit

PURPOSE

* To empty urinary collection bag

PROCEDURE

1. Assemble equipment:
   * disposable gloves
   * alcohol wipes
   * measuring device
   * paper towel
2. Wash hands and apply gloves.
3. Tell client what you plan to do.

4   Emptying a Drainage Unit

4. Place paper towel and measuring device on floor below drainage bag.
5. Open drain or spout and allow the urine to drain into measuring device (Figure 7–15A). Do not allow the tip of tubing to touch sides of the measuring device.
6. Close the drain and wipe it with the alcohol wipe. Replace it in the holder on the bag (Figure 7–15B).
7. Note the amount and color of urine. Empty urine into toilet. Wash and rinse the measuring device.
8. Remove gloves and wash hands.
9. Document amount of urine collected.

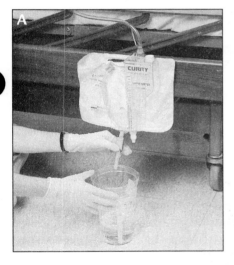 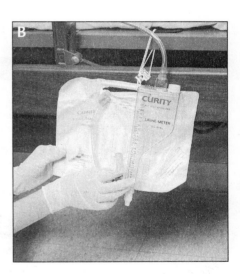

Figure 7–15   (A) Open the drain on the bottom of the collection bag. Allow the urine to drain into the measuring device. Note that the end of the drain is not touching the sides of the container. Wipe the drain off with alcohol before replacing. It is a good idea to use paper towels in case some urine is spilled. (B) Replace the drain in the slot in the bag.

bowel and bladder retraining
the process of restoring these lost functions to a client

Bowel and bladder retraining are important rehabilitation processes for clients with elimination dysfunction and incontinence. Some clients have lost all or part of their control and in some cases, the physician and the nurse may determine that bowel or bladder rehabilitation training may be useful to regain some or all of this control. Sometimes, incontinence can be prevented by offering the bedpan or urinal on a regular basis to the client.

For bowel training, the physician may order suppositories to stimulate the rectum to produce a bowel movement. The HCA may be asked to assist the client in inserting the suppository. The HCA should observe the client's ability to control his or her bowels in terms of how long the suppository is retained before a bowel movement occurs. Occasionally, enemas are ordered as part of bowel training and the HCA should check first with the supervisor to determine the agency's policy and procedure. States vary in the regulations concerning HCAs giving enemas. Commercially prepared enemas are usually approved for HCA use. Oil-retention enemas are also commercially prepared. The client should retain the oil in bed in a quiet position for as long as possible. Oil enemas work best if warmed first by soaking in warm water for 30 minutes. Refer to Procedure 5 for training and retraining bowels. Refer to Procedure 6 for how to give a rectal suppository. Refer to Procedure 7 for giving an enema.

CLIENT CARE PROCEDURE

5 Training and Retraining Bowels

PURPOSE

- To train a client to be continent of bowel movement
- To regulate a client to have regular bowel movements

NOTE: Constipation can result from illness, poor eating habits, drug therapy, and lack of exercise. Constipation causes the client added discomfort when it occurs in addition to other physical problems. An individualized bowel program is designed by the health care team for each client. For instance, one client can regulate the bowels by adding prune juice to the diet twice a day. Another client may need to drink daily prune juice and require a daily laxative and stool softener in addition.

Older clients can become overly "bowel conscious" and have a misconception of what normal elimination should be. The frequency of bowel movements may range from three times a day for one person to only once every two or three days for another. Therefore, the term constipation should not be used to describe a missed movement or two, but only the unusual retention of fecal matter along with infrequent or difficult passage of stony, hard stool.

Constipation is very often encountered among the elderly. If a client is unable to exercise and move about regularly, bowel action becomes sluggish. Sometimes medications, especially painkillers, can cause constipation. If a client has hemorrhoids, there may be a fear of pain and the client avoids trying to have a bowel movement. If a client does not have a bowel movement for a few days, he or she may develop an impaction, a large amount of hard stool in the lower colon or rectum. This is a very painful condition. If a client does develop an impaction, the nurse may have to remove it manually.

5   Training and Retraining Bowels

PROCEDURE

1. The health care team assesses prior habits of the client. If the client always had a bowel movement early in the morning, this is important to know in planning the retraining program.

2. A plan is designed and implemented. Important elements of the plan are:
   - high intake of fiber foods
   - adequate intake of liquids
   - regular exercise
   - toileting client at regular intervals
   - praise by aide at slightest progress of client
   - less reliance on laxatives and enemas
   - privacy for client during bowel movements

3. Follow bowel retraining program developed by the health care team. If the plan appears to be working, note success of program. If plan does not work, report that fact. It is also important to give some suggestions to the health care team of possible solutions for retraining the client.

6   Insertion of a Rectal Suppository

PURPOSE

- To relieve a client of constipation
- To make the client more comfortable

NOTE: A rectal suppository is a cone-shaped, easily melted, medicated mass that can readily be inserted into a client's rectum. Suppositories are usually stored in the client's refrigerator and are wrapped in foil. The suppository will melt once inserted into the warm environment of the rectum and colon. The suppository contains ingredients that once absorbed by the lining of the colon will give a stimulus to the colon to evacuate stool. It takes the suppository at least five to ten minutes to melt. It is important that the aide inform the client to wait a few minutes after the suppository is inserted before trying to have a bowel movement.

PROCEDURE

1. Assemble supplies:
   - rectal suppository
   - gloves
   - lubricant
   - protective pad or paper towels

CLIENT CARE PROCEDURE, *continued*

6   Insertion of a Rectal Suppository

2. Wash hands and apply gloves.

3. Tell client what you plan to do.

4. Open foil-wrapped suppository. Turn client on one side.

5. Lubricate gloved finger and insert suppository into rectum (see Figure 7–16). Push the suppository along the lining of the rectum with your index finger as far as your finger allows. Be careful not to insert suppository into the feces. The suppository needs to be next to the lining of the colon for it to be effective.

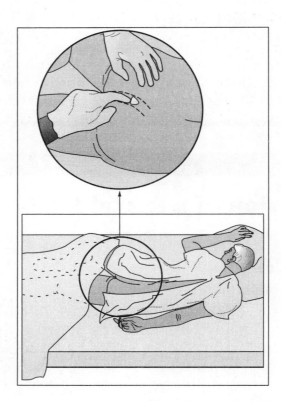

Figure 7–16   Carefully place the rectal suppository into the rectum about three inches on adult clients.

6. After ten minutes has passed, assist the client to the toilet or commode.

7. After client has had a bowel movement, assist client back to bed or chair.

8. Observe results of elimination.

9. Remove gloves and wash hands.

10. Record results. It is important to note color, consistency, and amount of stool.

7   Administering a Commercial Enema

PURPOSE

- To relieve the client of constipation
- To prepare client for diagnostic tests
- To make the client more comfortable

NOTE: An enema is the introduction of fluid into the rectum to remove feces and flatus (gas) from the rectum and colon.

Because enemas distend or dilate the rectum, the client may experience a feeling of urgency in the bowel; that is, a very strong need to empty the bowel as soon as possible.

Enemas can only be given on a doctor's orders.

The two commercially prepared enemas are the chemical (often referred to as Fleet®) and the oil-retention enemas. Oil-retention enemas are given to soften hard feces in the rectum and are usually followed by a soap solution enema.

PROCEDURE

1. Assemble supplies (see Figure 7–17)
   - gloves
   - commercial prepackaged enema
   - protective pad
   - bedpan (if client is bedridden)
   - toilet paper
   - lubrication jelly
2. Wash hands and put on gloves.

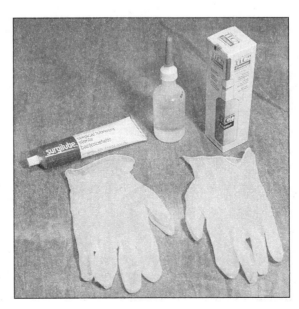

Figure 7–17 Equipment needed to administer a commercial enema

7 Administering a Commercial Enema

3. Tell client what you plan to do.

4. Provide for the client's comfort and privacy.

5. Have client turn onto the left side. Turn covers back to expose only the buttocks.

6. Remove cover on tip of enema. Apply extra lubricant to tip to ensure easy insertion.

7. Place protective pad underneath the client's buttocks.

8. Separate the buttocks and insert tip into rectum at least three inches. Tell client to take a deep breath and hold the solution as long as possible. Slowly squeeze the flexible plastic tube (see Figure 7–18). This forces the solution to flow evenly into the rectum.

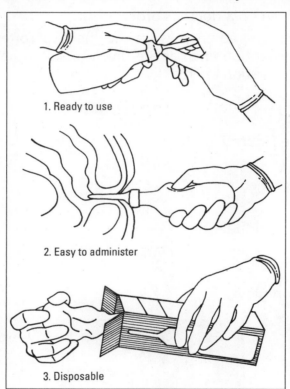

1. Ready to use

2. Easy to administer

3. Disposable

Figure 7–18 Administering a commercial enema. (Used with permission from C. B. Fleet Company, Inc., Lynchburg, VA)

9. Remove enema tip while holding the client's buttocks together.

10. Position client on bedpan, commode, or toilet.

11. After client has expelled feces and enema solution, assist the client in cleaning area around anus and buttocks.

12. Return client to comfortable position. It may be necessary to leave the protective pad in place until the effects of the enema are complete.

13. Remove gloves and wash hands.

14. Record results of enema as to color, amount, and consistency (for example, 10:00 AM, Fleet® enema given, good results, large, brown, formed stool).

Some of the areas to focus on for bowel training are:

1. Observe the bowel pattern by keeping a record of the time and character of each bowel movement.

2. Have the nurse check for fecal impaction, a collection of stool in the rectum which becomes larger than the anal opening.

3. Observe for signs of constipation or diarrhea.

4. Report any abdominal or rectal discomfort.

5. Establish regularity by offering the bedpan or bedside commode at regular times.

6. Administer bowel aides, such as suppositories or laxatives, as prescribed by the physician.

7. Offer a comfortable and private environment in which the client can move his or her bowels.

8. If the client is unsuccessful, offer a warm drink to stimulate the bowel movement.

Helpful Hint: Be sure not to communicate nonverbal messages, particularly facial expressions of disgust.

Adequate fluid intake is an important part of bowel training and to prevent constipation. Sometimes a special diet with increased fiber can be ordered by the physician to correct constipation. These diets encourage fresh raw and cooked vegetables and fruits, juices, whole grain products, protein-rich foods, bran and bran products, and lots of water. Bowel training can take up to eight weeks of client cooperation and consistent support from the HCA, the health care team, and the family.

bladder training training to restore the client's ability to control urination

Bladder training is most often ordered for clients who have problems with retention of urine resulting in incontinence. Retraining the bladder takes from six to eight weeks and emotional support may be a big factor in success. All members of the team, the client, and the family need to know what the training program is and how to play a role in the program. This is true for bowel training as well as bladder training. Figure 7–19 shows an example of a bladder retraining assessment sheet. The client's understanding, participation, and cooperation are vital to the success of the program. Refer to Procedure 8 for retraining the bladder.

Comp.# 1983 Page 1, Film 1, One Color, Punches on Left

BLADDER RETRAINING ASSESSMENT
(Reference tags: F315, F316)

CURRENT CLIENT STATUS

DIAGNOSIS_____ RESIDENT'S AGE_____

RECENT SURGERY? ☐ Yes ☐ No If Yes, date_____/_____/_____ and type_____

CURRENT MEDICATIONS (i.e., Diuretics, Psychotropics, etc.)_____
_____
_____

Mental Status and Ability to Communicate	Mobility Status	Vision Status	Right	Left
☐ Alert	☐ Independent	Adequate	☐	☐
☐ Aphasic	☐ Transfer/standing ability	Adequate w/aid	☐	☐
☐ Oriented x_____	☐ Wheelchair bound	Poor	☐	☐
☐ Disoriented	☐ Bed rest	Blind	☐	☐
☐ Depressed	☐ Contractures	**Hearing Status**	**Right**	**Left**
☐ Cooperative	☐ Other_____	Adequate	☐	☐
☐ Uncooperative	_____	Adequate w/aid	☐	☐
☐ Slow comprehension	_____	Poor	☐	☐
☐ Other_____	_____	Deaf	☐	☐

BLADDER ASSESSMENT

1. **LENGTH OF INCONTINENCE:** _____ Days _____ Months _____ Years

2. **REASON FOR INCONTINENCE (if known):** _____
   CATHETER: ☐ Yes ☐ No If Yes, specify type and size_____
   Date inserted _____/_____/_____ Reason for catheter _____

3. **USUAL VOIDING PATTERN:** Frequency_____ Amt./voiding_____ cc: /24 hrs._____ cc
   Pattern: ☐ Upon arising ☐ After meals ☐ No apparent pattern ☐ Night time only
   ☐ Other (specify)_____

4. **SYMPTOMS:** (Check all that apply)
   ☐ Voids often in small amounts ☐ Difficulty stopping stream ☐ Urgency
   ☐ Fills bladder/voids large amount ☐ Dribbles constantly ☐ Burning/Pain
   ☐ Unable to void ☐ Dribbles after voiding ☐ Edema
   ☐ Difficulty starting stream ☐ Dribbles while coughing ☐ Other (specify)_____

5. **HISTORY OF:** ☐ Urinary Disorders ☐ Bladder Disorders ☐ Kidney Disease ☐ Prostate Problems
   ☐ Neurological Disorders ☐ Fecal Impactions ☐ Other (specify)_____

6. **RELIEF AFTER VOIDING:** ☐ Complete ☐ Continued desire to void

7. **BLADDER DISTENDED:** ☐ Yes ☐ No **EMPTIED BY EXTERNAL STIMULI:** ☐ Yes ☐ No
   If Yes, Check: ☐ Kegel Exercises ☐ Warm water over perineum
   ☐ Other (specify)_____

8. **RESIDUAL URINE:** ☐ Yes ☐ No If Yes, Amount:_____ cc

9. **PERCEPTION OF NEED TO VOID:** ☐ Present ☐ Diminished ☐ Absent

10. **WELL HYDRATED:** ☐ Yes ☐ No **AVERAGE FLUID INTAKE (24 HRS)_____ cc**
    AVERAGE FLUID OUTPUT (24 HRS)_____ cc
    Fluids Preferred_____

NAME—Last	First	Middle	Attending Physician	Chart No.

CFS 6-10HH © 1992 Briggs Corporation, Des Moines, IA 50306 (800) 247-2343 Printed in U.S.A.

BLADDER RETRAINING ASSESSMENT
☐ Continued on Reverse

Figure 7–19 Bladder retraining assessment sheet *(continues)*

Comp.#1983 Page 2, Film 1, One Color, Backer for HH

EVALUATION FOR BLADDER RETRAINING POTENTIAL

☐ ABLE TO PARTICIPATE IN RETRAINING   EVALUATION PERIOD:_____ TO _____

PLAN:_____

_____

PROVIDE FLUIDS: **FLUIDS SHOULD BE SPACED AS FOLLOWS:**

_____ cc every 24 Hrs	☐ 7AM	☐ 11	☐ 3PM	☐ 7	☐ 11PM	☐ 3
_____ cc 7-3 shift	☐ 8	☐ 12N	☐ 4	☐ 8	☐ 12MN	☐ 4
_____ cc 3-11 shift	☐ 9	☐ 1PM	☐ 5	☐ 9	☐ 1AM	☐ 5
_____ cc 11-7 shift	☐ 10	☐ 2	☐ 6	☐ 10	☐ 2	☐ 6

OFFER NO FLUIDS AFTER _____ PM   TOILET FOR VOIDING EVERY ____ Hrs (Day and Evening) ____ Hrs (Night)
(Except as needed for medications)
RECORD RESULTS ON BLADDER RETRAINING RECORD.

☐ **UNABLE TO PARTICIPATE IN RETRAINING**

REASON:_____

_____

REEVALUATION DATE:_____

COMPLETED BY:_____   ___/___/___
                        Signature/Title   Date

BLADDER RETRAINING PROGRESS NOTES OR REEVALUATION NOTES

DATE	TIME	NOTES - ALL ENTRIES MUST BE SIGNED WITH NAME AND TITLE

NAME—Last	First	Middle	Attending Physician	Chart No.

BLADDER RETRAINING NOTES

Figure 7–19 *continued*

8 Retraining the Bladder

PURPOSE

- To regain bladder control

PROCEDURE

A home health aide must keep a record of how often and how much the client voids throughout the day and night for a few days. Once the client's voiding pattern is known, the nurse/supervisor can analyze the client's voiding record and formulate a schedule for the aide to follow. The schedule developed by the nurse will include regularly scheduled times for the aide to have the client drink a measured amount of fluid. After the client has drunk the liquid, the aide notes the time. Thirty minutes later, the aide toilets the client. The aide should encourage the client to void each time he or she is positioned on the commode or toilet. It is helpful at times to run water from the faucet to give the client an urge to void. Other methods include having the client apply light pressure to the bladder area to stimulate the urge to empty the bladder or having the client lean forward on the toilet to stimulate emptying the bladder. Remember that the client needs to be toileted at regular intervals to prevent accidents. The client needs consistent positive reinforcement to remain dry. At first it may be necessary to take the client to the bathroom every two hours; intervals may be lengthened as control is gained. A common cause of incontinence is delay in getting the client to the bathroom. It is of utmost importance to take the client to the bathroom on a regular time schedule. The plan also calls for the aide to maintain the client's fluid intake at about 2500 cc/day. The aide should encourage the client to wear regular underwear to enhance the client's self-esteem and to help him or her from reverting back to the previous incontinence habit.

Some of the areas to focus on in bladder retraining are:

1. Fluids should be encouraged in the daytime hours and restricted at night.

2. When offering the bedpan or commode, the client's positioning is important. Changing the height of the seat and hand rails can offer increasing comfort for the client. Men find it easier to urinate in a standing position.

3. Additional stimuli may encourage voiding (urinating) such as offering a glass of water, pouring water over the perineum, running water in the sink, bearing down, as is medically safe, to empty the bladder, and placing the client's hand in water.

4. The skin should be thoroughly cleaned on an incontinent client on a regular basis.

5. Caregivers should offer to assist the client to urinate on a regular schedule (every three to four hours).

Helpful Hint: Remember, patience is the key to motivating the client in bowel and bladder training.

6. Keep a careful record of the time and amount of urination on the intake and output sheets. Include any special problem areas and successful techniques for this client so other caregivers can offer consistent care. Refer to Procedure 9 for recording fluid intake and output.

CLIENT CARE PROCEDURE

9 Measuring and Recording Fluid Intake and Output

PURPOSE

- To identify food items that need to be measured for fluid intake
- To measure and record fluid intake and output accurately

NOTE: Intake is a measure of all the fluids or semiliquids that a person drinks. Output is all the fluid that passes out of the body. The abbreviation for measuring fluid intake and output is I&O. Figure 7–20 shows the fluids that should be included in the measurement of intake and output.

Measure for Intake	
ice	water
juices	pop
coffee	ice cream
yogurt	soup
Jell-o®	pudding
any other food that is liquid at room temperature	

Measure for Output	
vomitus (emesis)	liquid stools
urine	
blood or drainage from wounds	

Figure 7–20 Various fluids and substances are measured and recorded as intake and output.

PROCEDURE

1. Assemble supplies:
   - measuring cup or container for intake
   - large measuring container for output
2. Wash hands and apply gloves if measuring output.
3. Measure and record all liquids taken by the client. This includes all fluids taken with meals and between meals such as coffee, milk, fruit juices, beer, and water. Liquids are recorded in cubic centimeters, abbreviated cc (see Figure 7–21). Remember that 30 cc equals 1 ounce so if a client drank a can of pop that was 12 ounces, multiply 12 by 30 to equal 360 cc.
4. Ask the client to use a urinal or bedpan for all voiding. If the client can use the toilet, a special plastic "hat" can be placed in the toilet to collect the urine (see Figure 7–22). All urine must be collected so that it can be measured.
5. Pour urine from bedpan or urinal into a measuring device (see Figure 7–23). Record the amount. Always record output in cc.

CLIENT CARE PROCEDURE, *continued*

9 Measuring and Recording Fluid Intake and Output

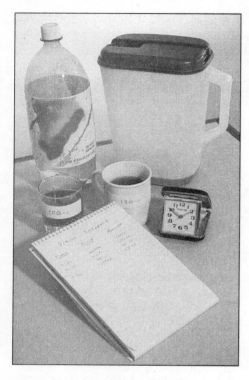

Figure 7–21 Measure the cubic centimeter (cc) capacity of commonly used glasses and cups. Record intake in cubic centimeters (cc) after the client has drunk the fluid.

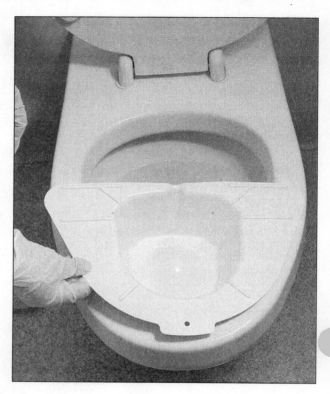

Figure 7–22 If a client's urine needs to be measured, a special toilet insert (potty hat) may be used to collect it.

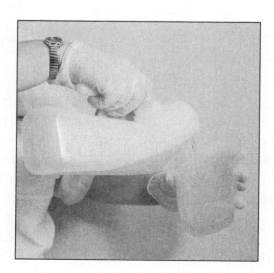

Figure 7–23 Urine can be measured with a special plastic container or a large measuring cup.

9 Measuring and Recording Fluid Intake and Output

6. Be sure to explain to the client how to keep exact records. The client must record the fluids at times when the aide is off duty.

7. Clean equipment after each use.

8. Remove gloves and wash hands.

NUTRITION

Providing proper nutrition to clients is always part of the HCA's client care. We discussed nutrition in Chapter 2 because approaches to nutrition are appropriate at different stages of the CVA recovery. During the acute phase, the HCA's part in the client's care is to observe and watch the sites of feeding tubes or intravenous feedings for signs of infection. These include any redness, swelling, discharge, or pain at the insertion area. The nurse is responsible for these more technical types of feedings. When swallowing is a problem, a **pureed diet** may be ordered. A pureed diet includes all the foods required, placed into a blender individually, and made into a semiliquid form. The food can then be swallowed more easily. The client who has had a stroke will be better able to eat the food, and still enjoy its taste.

pureed diet   a diet consisting of food blended or processed into a semiliquid form

Therapeutic (treatment) diets that may be ordered for these clients include:

1. Low sodium (restricted sodium) for clients with heart or kidney problems, or clients who retain fluids in body tissues. The average person should have less than 2,400 mg of sodium per day. Some restrictions are 500 mg/day.

2. Low fat or low cholesterol diet for clients with high cholesterol levels in their blood because they have a greater risk for heart attacks and/or strokes.

therapeutic (treatment) diets   diets specifically designed to be low in salt or sugar, high in carbohydrates, and so forth, to fit the particular needs of a client

Early in the recovery of a client who is learning to feed himself or herself again, the HCA may be doing the feeding at first. Later, as the OT begins to teach the client to use special feeding tools, the HCA assists with the feeding. Refer to Procedure 10 for assisting the client who can feed self and Procedure 11, feeding the dependent client.

CLIENT CARE PROCEDURE

10   Assisting the Client Who Can Feed Self

PURPOSE

- To provide proper nutrition for clients
- To provide food, based on client's condition, meeting standards of the food guide pyramid
- To provide a pleasurable experience for the client
- To encourage client to use adaptive devices for feeding

PROCEDURE

1. Assemble equipment:
   - Bedpan/urinal
   - Wash water
   - Oral hygiene items
   - Food
2. Offer bedpan/urinal or assist client to use the bathroom.
3. If permitted, elevate head of bed or assist client out of bed.
4. Clear overbed table and position in front of client (Figure 7–24). Remove sources of odors.
5. Provide water, soap, and towel to wash client's hands and face (Figure 7–25).
6. Assist with oral hygiene, if desired.

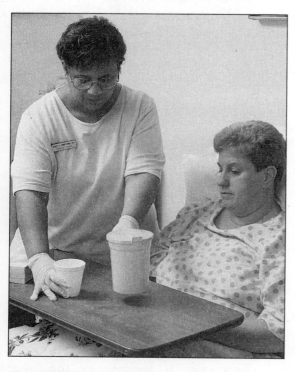

Figure 7–24   Clear off overbed table to make room for food tray.

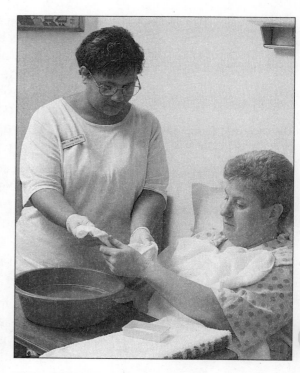

Figure 7–25   Give resident water to wash hands.

CLIENT CARE PROCEDURE , *continued*

10   Assisting the Client Who Can Feed Self

7. Wash your hands. Bring plate of food to overbed table.
8. Remove food as soon as client is finished. Be sure to note what the client has and has not eaten.
9. Record fluids on intake record, if necessary.
10. Push overbed table out of the way.
11. Help to perform oral hygiene to clean teeth, dentures, or mouth.

CLIENT CARE PROCEDURE

11   Feeding the Dependent Client

PURPOSE

- To provide proper nutrition for clients who are unable to feed themselves
- To provide suitable food, based on client's condition, meeting standards of the food guide pyramid
- To provide a pleasurable experience for the client
- To encourage client to use adaptive devices for feeding

PROCEDURE

1. Assemble equipment:
   - Bedpan/urinal
   - Wash water
   - Oral hygiene items
   - Food
2. Offer bedpan or urinal.
3. Provide oral hygiene if desired.
4. Remove unnecessary articles from the overbed table.
5. Elevate head of bed. Assist client into a sitting or upright position with head slightly bent forward. If client is out of bed, position client in chair in an upright position with feet flat on the floor.
6. Place napkin, bib, or towel under client's chin (Figure 7–26).

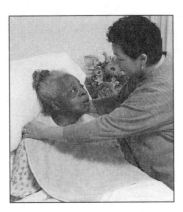

Figure 7–26   Place a towel or bed protector under the resident's chin.

11   Feeding the Dependent Client

7. Wash hands.

8. Place plate of food on the overbed table. Sit down facing the client so you are at eye level. The environment should be quiet and calm.

9. Holding spoon at right angle:

   - Give solid foods from tip of spoon (Figure 7–27).
   - Alternate solids and liquids.
   - Rotate the offerings of food to give variety.
   - Describe or show client what kind of food you are giving.
   - Direct food to unaffected side of mouth and check for food stored in affected side.
   - Test hot foods by dropping a small amount on the inside of your wrist before feeding them to the client.
   - Never blow on the client's food to cool it.
   - Never taste the client's food.
   - Do not hurry the meal.

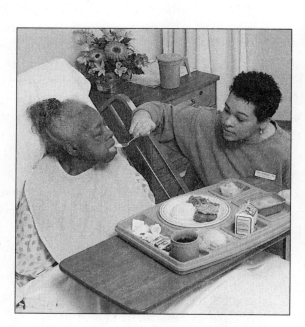

Figure 7–27   Give solid foods from the tip of the spoon

10. Allow client to hold bread or assist to the extent possible.

11. Use napkin to wipe client's mouth as often as necessary.

12. Remove food as soon as client is finished. Be sure to note what the client has and has not eaten.

13. Provide oral hygiene.

11 Feeding the Dependent Client

14. Record fluids on intake record, if necessary.
15. Push overbed table out of the way.
16. Wash hands.

Feeding is only part of the HCA's responsibility in caring for the client's nutrition. Other duties include:

- understanding special therapeutic diets, such as low sodium or low cholesterol
- assisting with the planning of meals to provide a balanced diet
- purchasing foods if time permits, or assisting the client and family to shop and to read food labels properly
- preparing meals when time permits and the care plan includes such duties
- observing, reporting, and recording the client's nutritional level

When the HCA is with the client and family every day or living in all the time, there is more time for such tasks. The time the HCA has is the determining factor in the extra duties of purchasing and preparing meals. When this is not possible, but there is still a problem with offering nutritious meals, a meal plan may be necessary, such as a food service which delivers meals to the home. The most important aspect is the planning because there are factors that affect the nutrition levels of every client.

For the HCA to be sure the client is getting proper nutrition, it may be necessary to have a dietitian consult. The client may need to eat a food supplement such as Ensure® or other high-protein drinks. Weighing the client on a weekly basis is a good way to determine if proper nutrition is being given.

Choking may be a problem for clients who have had a stroke because of poor swallowing ability. Foods should not be dry, and meats are especially dangerous if not chopped or cut into small bites.

Fluid intake is always important to provide the body with adequate hydration. These clients frequently do not drink enough fluids. Older persons need two to three quarts of fluid per day. The HCA should:

- be sure the client is not the exception and on restricted fluids
- prepare and offer fresh water in a pitcher or glass frequently
- assist the client with drinking if necessary (use straws and special cups or glasses)
- find out what liquids the client likes and dislikes

HOME ENVIRONMENT

Safety of the home environment is discussed in Chapter 9. However, that is only one aspect of the home environment that is important in client care of the stroke victim. Other important areas include maintaining a healthy home for these special clients in which they can be rehabilitated and finally adapt to caring for themselves as much as possible. The therapists play a part in determining how the home should be set up to accommodate any assistive devices the client uses for ambulation.

Home maintenance may be a function the HCA provides in the home for the client needing rehabilitation. If the caretaker of the home is the client, other members of the family may not be familiar with caring for the home and all that may involve. The role the HCA plays in maintaining a healthy and clean environment for the client may include light housekeeping, laundry, shopping, and meal service. Figure 7–28 shows the HCA cleaning to maintain a healthy environment.

A clean home offers less risk of infection and accidents and promotes a comfortable surrounding for the client. Many times, the home maintenance duties involve the client's bedroom, the kitchen, and the bathroom areas. If the HCA is not in the home for long periods of time, it is important that he or she sets up a schedule with other team members and caregivers so that household tasks can be distributed. The following are some important areas to remember in home maintenance:

1. Keep the home organized and tidy.
2. Keep a shopping list so that cleaning supplies and laundry supplies are available.
3. Kitchen floors should be kept clean of spills and crumbs.
4. Air the client's room (if weather permits) to reduce infection risk.

home maintenance keeping the home a safe and healthy environment

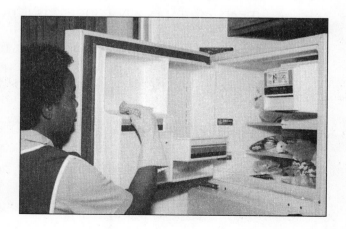

Figure 7–28 Clean spills up immediately.

5. Properly clean and store food in the kitchen to create an aseptic environment.
6. Check the cupboards for food and keep a shopping list.
7. Keep the bathroom and kitchen clean to avoid the spread of microorganisms.
8. Clean tubs, sinks, and shower every day.
9. Keep bathroom floors free of spills to avoid accidents.
10. Delegate someone in the family to keep a good supply of linens for the client's daily use.

The client at home functions best if the daily schedule is set in an established routine and followed day to day. Changes of any type are especially troublesome. Going out of the home for meals or visits should not be attempted until the client is comfortable and when special equipment can be taken along without embarrassment.

The client will let the family and HCA know if and when outside activity is desired. Until then, the client should get up and dress every morning and follow as normal a routine as possible. The home environment should be comfortable, but not revolve around the client's disabilities.

REPOSITIONING THE CLIENT

Repositioning the client is an important procedure, both for client comfort and to prevent contractures. Good body alignment for the client is very important. The back should be straight and in alignment during transfers and while the client is in any position. The HCA should know if there are any problems the client has or positions which are not appropriate. When turning the client, the drawsheet should be used to prevent friction on the skin. Shearing, or forcing the skin to move in an opposite direction, causes skin breakdown and should be avoided. Procedures 12, 13, 14, and 15 show how to correctly position the client.

CLIENT CARE PROCEDURE

12   Positioning the Client in Supine Position

PURPOSE

- To make the client more comfortable
- Assist the body to function more efficiently

12   Positioning the Client in Supine Position

PROCEDURE

1. Wash your hands.
2. Tell client what you plan to do.
3. Place pillow under the client's head about two inches above the level of the bed. the pillow should extend slightly under the shoulders (see Figure 7–29).

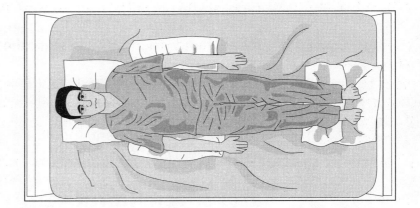

Figure 7–29   A client in supine position. The head may be elevated slightly with a pillow and the arms supported with pillows for comfort. A pillow is placed under the feet to prevent pressure on the heels.

4. Have client's arms extend straight out with palms of the hands flat on the bed. The arms can be supported by pillows or covered foam pads placed under the forearms, extending from just above the elbows to the ends of the fingers.
5. Place a small pillow or rolled towel along the side of the client's thighs and tuck part of the support under the thigh, ensuring that it is smooth. This maintains alignment of the hips and thighs and helps prevent the hips from rotating outward or externally.
6. Place a pillow under the back of the ankle to relieve pressure on the heels.
7. Wash your hands.
8. Document the time, position change, and the client's reaction.

13   Positioning the Client in Lateral Side-laying Position

PURPOSE

- To provide client comfort
- To relieve pressure on body parts

13 Positioning the Client in Lateral Side-laying Position

PROCEDURE

1. Wash your hands.
2. Tell client what you plan to do.
3. Go to the side of the bed opposite the direction from which you are planning to turn the client.
4. Cross the client's arms over the chest. Place your arm under the client's neck and shoulders. Place your other arm under the client's midback. Move the upper part of the client's body toward you.
5. Place one arm under the client's waist and the other under the thighs. Move the lower part of the client's body toward you.
6. Turn client to opposite side. Pull shoulder that is touching the bed slightly toward you. Pull buttock that is touching the bed slightly toward you. Place pillow under back and buttocks. Place bottom leg in extension and flex upper leg. Place small folded blanket or pillow between the upper and lower legs.
7. Place pillow under the client's head. Rotate the upper arm to bring it up to the pillow with the palm facing up. Place the other arm on a pillow that extends from above the elbow to the fingers. Extend the fingers.
8. Check the client's position to see if the body is in good vertical alignment (see Figure 7–30).

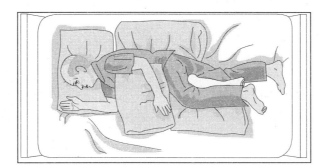

Figure 7–30   Lateral/side-laying position

9. Wash your hands.
10. Document time, change of position, and client's reaction.

14 Positioning the Client in Prone Position

PURPOSE

- To relieve pressure on body parts.
- To provide client comfort

CLIENT CARE PROCEDURE, *continued*

14   Positioning the Client in Prone Position

NOTE: Most elderly clients are not able to lie on their stomachs and do not like to be in this position for long periods of time. Before turning a dependent client to the prone position, make sure client's arms are straight down at sides to avoid injury while turning. Never leave an older client in this position for more than 15 to 20 minutes.

PROCEDURE

1. Wash your hands.
2. Tell client what you plan to do.
3. Turn client on abdomen. Check to see if spine is straight and face is turned to one side or the other.
4. Legs should be extended and arms flexed and brought up to either side of head.
5. A small pillow can be placed under the abdomen, especially for women, because this reduces pressure against their breasts. An alternate method is to roll a small towel and place it under the shoulders to reduce pressure.
6. Place another pillow under lower legs to prevent pressure on toes (see Figure 7–31). Client can also be moved to foot of bed so that the feet extend over the mattress.

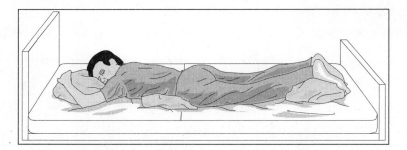

Figure 7–31   Prone position

7. Wash your hands.
8. Document time, position change, and client's reaction.

CLIENT CARE PROCEDURE

15   Positioning the Client in Fowler's Position

PURPOSE

- To provide client comfort
- To aid in breathing
- To position client so that he or she can engage in activities such as eating, reading, watching television, or visiting with a family member or friend.

15   Positioning the Client in Fowler's Position

NOTE: If the client is weak or frail, the sitting position may be hard for him or her to maintain. Support the client with pillows to help maintain the sitting position.

PROCEDURE

1. Wash your hands.
2. Tell the client what you plan to do.
3. Check to see if the client is supine and legs are straight and that he or she is in the middle of the bed.
4. Support client's head and neck with one, two, or three pillows. If client has a hospital bed, raise bed to a 45-degree angle.
5. Knees may be flexed and supported with small pillows (see Figure 7–32).

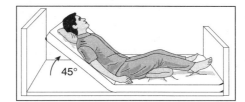

Figure 7–32   Fowler's position

6. Pillows may be placed under each arm from elbows to fingertips to support shoulders.
7. Place pillow or padded footboard against feet.
8. Wash your hands.
9. Document time, position change, and client's reaction.

The client's posture and the HCA's posture are both important. Many clients can help with the moving process. However, the HCA may be repositioning clients who cannot help. In this case, it may require two persons to perform the positioning procedure. The family caregiver may assist the HCA when necessary. The HCA should have a plan for positioning the client and have pillows and other devices ready before beginning the procedure. Before moving the client, the HCA should review the principles of body mechanics which include:

- correct posture to make lifting, pulling, and pushing easier (Fig. 7–33A and B)
- keeping the back straight and using the thigh muscles, not the back muscles (Figure 7–34)
- turn in pivoting motion, not from the waist (Figure 7–35A and B)

- holding heavy objects close to the body (Figure 7–36)
- pushing, pulling, or rolling rather than lifting
- keeping feet approximately twelve inches apart for proper body support (Figure 7–37)
- using verbal signals to let the client and other workers know when the move is to be made

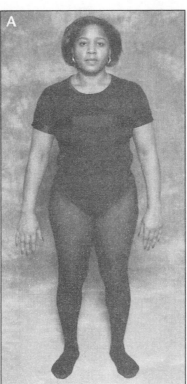

Figure 7–33 Correct standing position—A. Front view, B. Side view

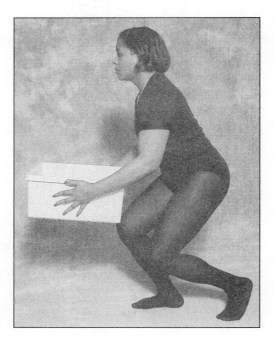

Figure 7–34 The correct way to maintain balance when picking up an object is to bend from the hips and knees.

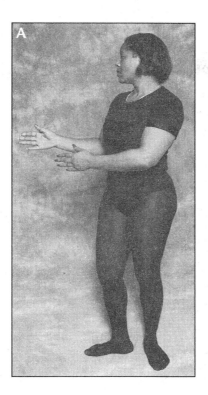 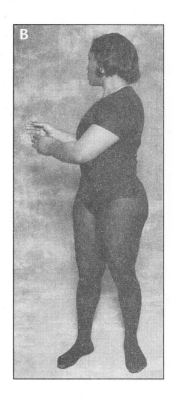

Figure 7–35   A. Pivot instead of twisting—B. Avoid twisting the body

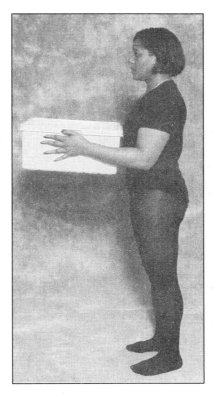

Figure 7–36   Hold objects close to the body

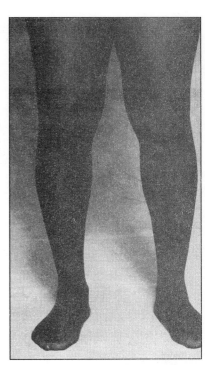

Figure 7–37   Keep feet apart

Repositioning clients is done when they are in bed and when they are sitting in chairs. Proper repositioning prevents complications, such as pressure sores and body deformities. The following are general guidelines for lifting and moving clients.

1. The HCA should know special considerations about the client before beginning and discuss repositioning with the supervisor.

2. Have a written plan so that positions can be varied during a 24 hour period.

3. Always tell the client what will be done so that the client can help as much as possible if the treatment plan permits.

4. Be careful not to touch painful areas.

5. Be gentle and use slow, smooth movements. Stop if there is pain.

6. Allow the client periods of rest during the procedure if it becomes necessary.

Supportive devices may be needed to keep the body in proper alignment. Some of these devices may include footboards to prevent foot drop, special foot devices to help maintain foot position (Figure 7–38), bedboards to make the mattress firm, trochanter rolls to prevent the hips and legs from turning outward (Figure 7–39), hand rolls to prevent contractures of the hands and wrists, and bed cradles to keep the linens off of the feet (Figure 7–40).

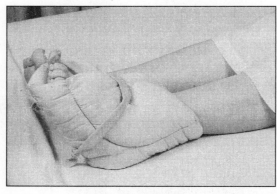

Figure 7–38   Special foot devices keep the foot in the correct position

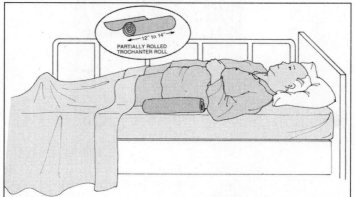

Figure 7–39   Trochanter roll in place

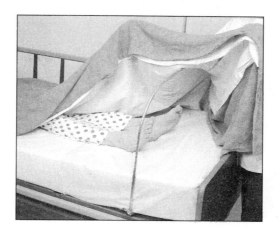

Figure 7–40 A bed cradle keeps sheets from putting pressure on the feet.

When positioning the client, the HCA will need several pillows (usually three or four). They can be of various sizes to support the head or the back and to keep the client from rolling off the side. Rolled towels or blankets can be used in the home between the legs or ankles and between bones to prevent friction. They also can be used as trochanter rolls. Footboards can be purchased or blankets and boxes placed at the foot of the bed. All clients who are on repositioning programs should have turning sheets and/or draw sheets. Turning schedules usually provide client position changes at least every two hours in a systematic way.

SKIN CARE

pressure ulcers open sores which occur when undue pressure or friction is applied to the skin for hours at a time

Skin care is given to rehabilitation clients to prevent breakdown of the skin which could lead to **pressure ulcers**. When there is pressure, shearing, or friction on the skin, breakdown occurs. Because clients requiring rehabilitation have impaired mobility, their risk is higher for decubitus ulcers. Other contributing factors may include: lack of cleanliness, moisture (such as perspiration or urine), incontinence, and soap left on the skin. The skin breaks down in four stages:

Stage I: Redness lasting longer than 30 minutes after pressure is removed. The area may be warm to the touch.

Stage II: The skin is reddened and has a blister or broken area on the surface.

Stage III: Layers of the skin have been destroyed and may or may not be infected.

Stage IV: Skin is gone and the ulcer is deep into the muscle and bone.

Figure 7–41A–D shows the four stages of skin breakdown. Figure 7–42 shows the most common sites for skin breakdown.

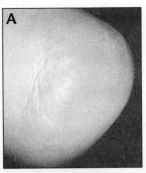

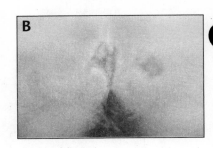

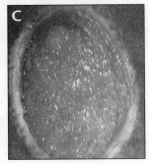

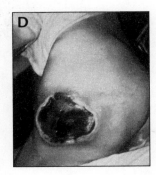

Figure 7–41   A. First indication of tissue ischemia (Stage I) is redness and heat over a pressure point such as this heel.
B. Stage II is marked by destruction of the epidermis and partial destruction of the dermis. Photo shows coccygeal (sacrum) area.
C. In Stage III, all layers of skin have been destroyed and deep crater has been formed. Photo shows right hip.
D. In Stage IV, skin is gone and ulcer is deep into muscle and bone. Courtesy of Emory University Hospital, Atlanta, GA.)

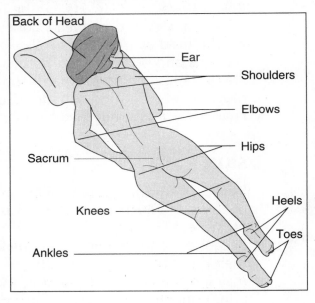

Figure 7–42   Most common sites of skin breakdown

Seven ways to prevent skin breakdown are:

1.   Remove pressure from bony areas.
2.   Massage the skin surrounding the area.
3.   Keep skin clean and dry.
4.   Keep repositioning the client.
5.   Remove urine and feces from the skin promptly.
6.   Pat skin dry instead of rubbing.
7.   Give back massages.

The client's skin should be observed regularly and accurately, especially at pressure points (Figure 7–43). The HCA should report any changes in the skin, such as redness, heat, tenderness, or blisters immediately. The HCA should keep a record of changing the position of the client. Figure 7–44 is an example of a chart used to record position changes. Incontinent clients should be checked for dryness frequently (every one to two hours) and measures taken to keep urine and feces off the skin by use of protective pads or briefs. Disposable briefs should be changed frequently. Preventative devices can be used to prevent skin breakdown, such as specialty beds, specialty mattresses, sheepskin heel and elbow protectors, and bed cradles.

Refer to Procedure 16 for special skin care and pressure sores.

> **Helpful Hint:** The HCA should always report suspicious skin areas to the supervisor immediately to protect the client, the agency, and himself or herself.

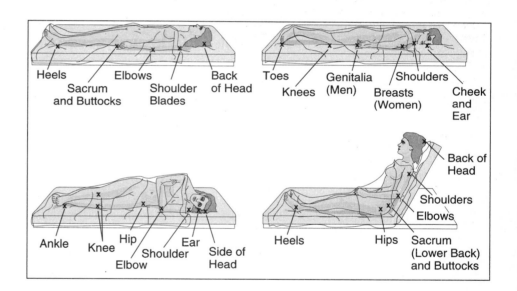

Figure 7–43 Possible pressure points

FRAMINGHAM HOME POSITION-CHANGE BEDSIDE RECORD							
NAME Smith, Emily					ROOM NUMBER 118B		
DATE	TIME	POSIT.	SIGNA.	DATE	TIME	POSIT.	SIGNA.
4/17	7 AM	Dorsal Recombent	JH.				
	9 AM	Left Sims	JH.				
	11 AM	Prone	JH.				

Figure 7–44 The position change record should be kept at the bedside for convenience.

CLIENT CARE PROCEDURE

16 Special Skin Care and Pressure Sores

PURPOSE

- To prevent skin breakdown resulting from pressure and skin irritations
- To use preventative devices
- To prevent friction resulting from skin being in contact with skin or bed linens

NOTE: Certain clients are at risk for the development of pressure areas leading to sores. Clients at risk are bedridden: they may be obese, very thin, diabetic, paralyzed, and/or malnourished. The HCA's role is mainly in the prevention of pressure sore development. Once a pressure sore has developed, the nurse then comes to the client's home to treat the open area.

ASSISTIVE DEVICES TO PREVENT PRESSURE SORES

1. Air mattress—This is a mattress filled with air. It works by continuously changing the pressure areas on the client's back. One can improvise with an air mattress designed for camping instead of buying a medical air mattress.
2. Egg crate mattress—This is a mattress made from foam rubber molded into an egg crate pattern. Egg crate mattresses are inexpensive and effective in reducing pressure on the skin. One can also purchase a seat for the client to sit on during the day when up in a chair.
3. Water mattress—This is similar to a regular water mattress used in the home. The mattress is effective in reducing pressure on the skin but causes problems when transferring clients in and out of bed.
4. Gel foam cushion—This is a special cushion filled with a special solution or gel. The cushion is effective in the prevention of pressure sores for the client who sits in a wheelchair for long periods of time.
5. Sheepskin or lamb's wool pads for elbows and heels—Lamb's wool pads prevent pressure sores by acting as a barrier between the client's skin and the sheets.
6. Bed cradle—This is a device to keep linens off the client's legs and feet. In the home, an aide can substitute a box or other device to keep linens off the legs and feet.

SPECIAL CARE TO PREVENT PRESSURE SORES

1. Change client's position at least every two hours to reduce pressure on any one area.
2. As quickly as possible, remove feces, urine, or moisture of any kind that might be irritating to the skin.
3. Encourage clients who sit in chairs or wheelchairs to raise themselves or change position every 15 minutes to relieve pressure.
4. Encourage client to eat a high-protein diet (if allowed by the physician) and to drink adequate amounts of fluids.
5. Keep bed linens clean, dry, and wrinkle-free.
6. When bathing clients, use soap sparingly because soap drys skin. Keep skin well lubricated.

16   Special Skin Care and Pressure Sores

7. Watch for skin irritation when applying braces and splints.

8. At the first sign of a reddened area, gently massage area around the spot. Report observations to the nurse or supervisor immediately.

The HCA should follow the guidelines set down by the agency for special skin care programs. Cleanliness is the main objective, along with careful observation and documentation. The HCA can apply special creams and ointments as directed by the nurse or supervisor and stimulate circulation in the client's back, buttocks, and bony areas through massage.

ASSISTING WITH DRESSING THE CLIENT

Assistance with dressing the client is frequently required with rehabilitation clients. There are many dressing aids on the market which are listed in the equipment section of this module. The client should always be encouraged to do as much as possible according to the physician's orders, the nursing care plan, and the client's limitations. Clients should be encouraged not to wear pajamas during the day, but rather to dress in their clothes to encourage a feeling of participation in a normal life.

Bedbound clients, of course, will have to be dressed or assisted to dress by the HCA. Bedbound clients should be in hospital gowns if possible to make the dressing and undressing easier on the workers. Bedclothes that are easily changed are best. However, even clients who are bedbound can select their clothes and do as much self-care as possible.

Before assisting the clients in dressing, the HCA should have the client select their clothes for the day. This gives the client a feeling of control and increases self-esteem. Clothing should be clean and neat, and not loose fitting or present a problem in safety for the client who has a physical limitation. Refer to Procedure 17 for dressing and undressing the client.

Helpful Hint: It sometimes takes great patience on the part of the person assisting the client. Let the client have plenty of time without feeling rushed.

17   Dressing and Undressing the Client

PURPOSE

- To keep the client clean and comfortable
- To increase the client's self-image and well-being
- To reduce client's discomfort and reduce his or her risk of strain or injury

NOTE: Do not allow the client to remain in nightclothes during the day (unless the case manager states it is permitted). The client needs to know that it is daytime and to dress accordingly.

PROCEDURE

1. Wash your hands and tell the client what you plan to do.
2. Assemble clean clothing:
   - undergarments
   - outergarments—let clients select their own, if possible
   - stockings and shoes
3. If client is able, help him or her to sit at the edge of the bed and dangle the legs. If the client is too weak to sit up, have him or her lie flat on the bed. Place a sheet or robe over the client to avoid embarrassment or chilling.
4. Assist the client in putting on undergarments. If the client has a weak leg, place weak leg in first, then the other leg. Put on outergarments in the same manner. If client can stand, pull the pants or slacks up to the waist. If the client must remain on the bed, ask the client to press his or her heels into the bed and raise the buttocks. While the client is in this position, quickly slide the pants or slacks up to the waist. Assist the client as necessary. Slacks with elastic waists are preferred as they go on easier than pants with zippers and buttons. Cotton jogging suits are becoming a very popular option for disabled or elderly clients. They are warm, easy to get off and on, and attractive. They also launder easily.
5. To dress the client in a shirt, slip, or dress, help the client place the weak arm into the sleeve first (Figure 7–45A), then the strong arm. If the dress or shirt needs to go over the head, help client place both arms into the armholes and then slip the neck of the garment over the client's head.

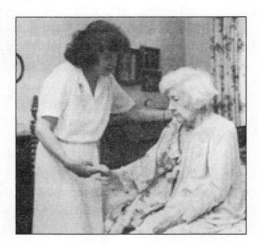

Figure 7–45A   Place weak arm into sleeve first, followed by the strong arm.

17 Dressing and Undressing the Client

6. To put on socks or stockings, turn each sock down to the toe end. Slide client's toe into place, and with one arm on each side of leg, pull the sock or stocking up (Figure 7–45B). Make sure socks are smooth over the feet and legs. Put on shoes if client is to remain out of bed. Let client assist as much as possible.

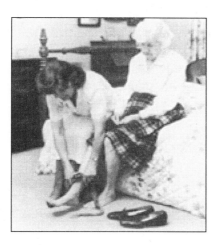

Figure 7–45B   Roll stocking down to the toe, then put on the foot.

7. To undress the client, simply reverse the instructions for dressing. If the client has a weak arm or leg, undress the weak limb last.
8. Wash hands.

RANGE OF MOTION

Range of motion exercises are done to prevent joint contractures and maintain or increase joint mobility. The HCA who has been trained to do ROM exercises performs this procedure in one of the following four ways:

1. Passive ROM, in which the client does not participate and movements are done by the HCA completely.
2. Active-assistive ROM, in which the client participates but still requires the HCA's assistance.
3. Active ROM, in which the client performs all of the movements and the HCA observes and records the procedure.
4. Resistive ROM, in which the client performs the movements with weights.

   Refer to Procedure 17 for range of motion exercises.

18 Performing Passive Range of Motion Exercises

PURPOSE

- To increase muscle tone and strength in the client's body
- To restore function to injured parts of the body
- To prevent joint stiffness and contractures

NOTE: Do not perform the exercises until you have received instructions specific for your client's joints. When possible, support the extremity above and below the joints being exercised. If the client shows pain or discomfort, stop the exercise and document it. The head can be exercised if specifically ordered by the physical therapist. Exercises can be done in bed or in the chair. It is important to keep the client covered or clothed to prevent unnecessary exposure during the procedure.

PROCEDURE

1. Wash your hands.
2. Read any special instructions for the exercises for your client.
3. Tell client what you plan to do. Ask client to assist as much as possible.
4. Exercise the shoulder—Supporting the upper and lower arms, exercise the shoulder joint. Abduct (away from the body) the entire arm out at right angles to the body (Figure 7–46A). Then adduct the arm (bring back to the midline of the body) to the center of the client's body (Figure 7–46B).
5. Exercise the elbow—Bend elbow, keeping the arm close to the body. Bring the fingers up to touch the shoulder (Figure 7–47A). Lower the fingers down to touch the bed (Figure 7–47B).

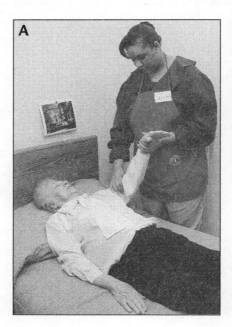
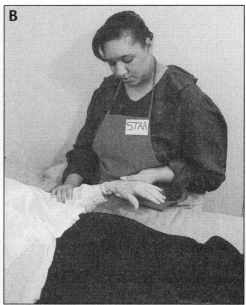

Figure 7–46 Exercising the shoulder joint

18 Performing Passive Range of Motion Exercises

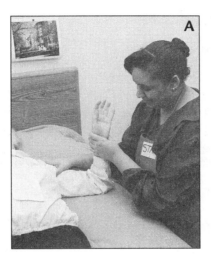
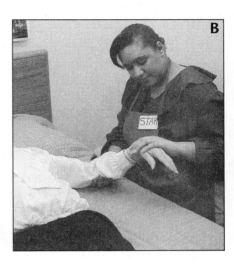

Figure 7–47 Exercising the elbow

6. Exercise the forearm—Bring the arm out to the side. Rest it on the bed. Take the client's hand and rotate the arm, palm up and palm down (Figure 7–48A and B).

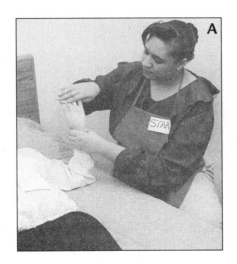
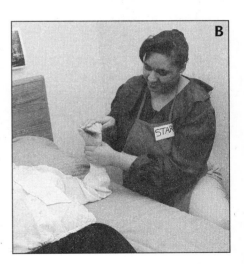

Figure 7–48 Exercising the forearm

7. Exercise the wrist and fingers—Take the client's hand and move the hand forward and back (Figure 7–49A and B). Move the hand from side to side. Curl the client's fingers and straighten them (Figure 7–49C and D). Spread the fingers apart and rotate the thumb. Touch all fingers to thumb (Figure 7–49E).

8. Exercise the knee and hip—Keep the client lying on his or her back. Bend the knee and raise it to the chest (Figure 7–50). Bring the leg out to the side and back. Cross one leg over the other. Allow the leg to rest on the bed with the knee straight and the heel resting on the bed. Rotate the leg inward and outward.

18 Performing Passive Range of Motion Exercises

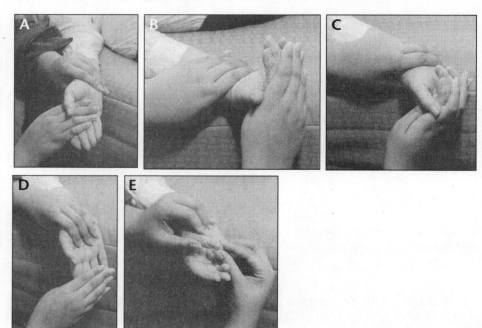

Figure 7–49 Exercising the wrist and fingers

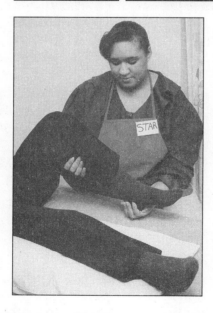

Figure 7–50 Exercising the knee and hip

9. Exercise the ankle—Bend client's knee slightly and support lower leg with one hand. With the other hand, bend client's foot downward (plantar flexion) and then bend client's foot toward the body (dorsiflexion) (Figure 7–51A and B). With client's legs extended on the bed, place both hands on the client's foot and move foot inward and then outward.

10. Exercise the toes—Bend (flexion) and straighten (extension) each toe. Perform abduction and adduction with each toe as you did with the fingers.

11. Move to the client's other side and repeat movements for each joint.

18 Performing Passive Range of Motion Exercises

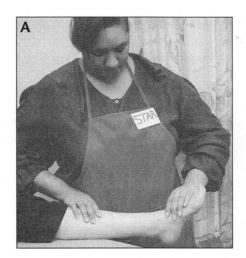 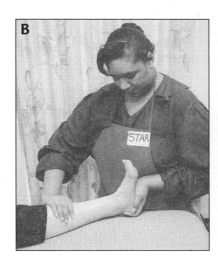

Figure 7–51 Exercising the ankle and foot

12. Wash hands.

13. Document the completion of the exercises and the client's reactions.

ROM exercises are usually performed with the client in bed, but can be done with the client standing. The benefits to the client of performing ROM exercises are to keep the muscles strong and the joints working, prevent deformities and spasticity, promote blood circulation, improve mobility and coordination, and enhance the client's self-esteem. In some cases, the PT Assistant or the OT perform the ROM exercises for the client.

ROM exercises are performed as prescribed in the treatment plan and described in the care plan, and are usually done during or after the bath and again later in the day. Some clients need to perform ROM exercises as often as every four hours. The following are guidelines to follow for ROM exercises.

1. The HCA should always check the care plan and/or supervisor's instructions for the client's **functional limitation**.

2. Each exercise should be done five times unless otherwise instructed.

3. The joints to be exercised should be specifically ordered.

4. When appropriate, the HCA should begin at the head and work toward the feet in an organized manner.

5. The HCA should be careful not to expose the client during the exercise (put underpants or pajama bottoms on the client).

6. The HCA should encourage the client to do as much as he or she can if that is the order.

functional limitation the client's level of ambulation and activity

7. The HCA should never force an extremity past a comfortable point.

8. If the client complains of pain, the HCA should stop the exercise and report to the supervisor.

9. The arm or leg being exercised should be supported.

10. The HCA should use slow, smooth, gentle movements.

11. If the joint or extremity appears to be swollen, red, or painful, the HCA should stop and report to the supervisor.

12. If the client refuses to do the exercises, the HCA should report immediately to the supervisor.

13. The HCA should document what exercises were done, the time, any observations, and how the client responded.

SUMMARY

The special skills and procedures required to care for a client who has had a stroke are important to the outcome of the case. It is the HCA who does most of the hands-on care and interacts on a visit-to-visit basis with the client. All the procedures in this chapter should be part of the specially trained HCA's abilities. The success or failure of these procedures could have far-reaching implications for the client down the road of recovery.

CASE STUDY

Your post-CVA client is bedridden and requires home care around the clock. He has a urinary catheter, is incontinent of stool, and must be fed. You have agreed to twelve-hour shifts in which the family cares for the client the other twelve hours of every day. What important HCA procedures would the family be expected to perform and how can you be supportive of them?

REVIEW QUESTIONS

1. Home maintenance usually includes _____ , _____ , _____ , and _____ .

2. The _____ will determine the setup of the home to accommodate assistive devices.

3. Which gait requires strong upper arms and probably is not appropriate for post-stroke clients?

4. The urinary draining bag should:

   a. be higher than the client

   b. never be emptied by the aide

   c. kept clean of feces

   d. be cleaned once a week

5. A diet high in fiber would not necessarily include:

   a. fresh vegetables

   b. raw vegetables

   c. bran products

   d. Jell-O®

6. Fresh water is important because it:

   a. lowers pain

   b. increases fluid level

   c. stimulates urination

   d. stimulates appetite

7. True or False? ADLs are different for everyone.

8. True or False? The process of self-care is long and difficult for persons who have suffered a stroke.

9. True or False? Successful preventative measures will leave the client with no deformities.

10. True or False? HCAs are not a part of self-care.

11. Unscramble the following key term from the chapter: urettecaphi tdies _____ _____

Client/Family Education

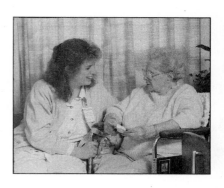

OBJECTIVES

Upon reading this chapter and completing the review questions, the home care aide should be able to:

1. Recognize the nurse's educational plan and the factors for success.

2. Motivate and encourage the client/family to respond to the teaching elements.

3. Describe the education process and the HCA's role.

KEY TERMS

compliance
education plan
empower

motivator
reinforce

INTRODUCTION

In caring for a client who has had a stroke, it is vital that the rehabilitation process be a team effort. In Chapter 4, we described the multidisciplinary team. The home health care team consists of all trained personnel involved in the client's day-to-day care and treatment. There are two additional team members who play the greatest part in the success or failure of the rehabilitation of the client: the client himself or herself and the family. Very few rehabilitation programs would last without the full cooperation and participation of the client and his or her family. This is accomplished through a comprehensive education plan which, in the case of the client who has had a CVA, is developed by the therapists, the physician, and the nurse. The HCA also has a part to play in the education plan because he or she spends more time with the client and family than the other members of the

motivator a person who encourages another

team. The HCA is in the best position to observe how the education plan is working. The HCA will be the **motivator,** or person who encourages or motivates the client to do as much as possible to stay healthy and well.

THE EDUCATION PLAN

education plan the day-to-day organization and process of the client/family teaching prepared by the nurse

It is important for the HCA to understand the importance of the **education plan** and to keep current on its progress or lack of progress. Also, the HCA who specializes in caring for clients who have had a stroke and require rehabilitation must accept a responsibility to meet the following four main goals of client/family education:

1. Always have a clear understanding of the client's day-to-day condition, and how that is reflected in the documentation and HCA and nursing care plans.
2. Observing and reporting any family needs, questions, and problems to the supervisor by keeping channels of communication open at all times.
3. Knowing and understanding which educational and teaching content the therapist and/or nurse on the case are using for the client/family so there is consistent follow-up to their instructions.
4. Acting as a professional role model and setting a good example for the client and family as procedures and tasks are performed from day to day.

Because the health care team cannot be in the home 24 hours a day, the continuation of the rehabilitation process must be performed by the family. Therefore, the education provided to give the client and family the knowledge and skills to continue the care is quite important. The ultimate goal of home health care is to return the client to the highest level of functioning. Without proper education, this is not possible.

Helpful Hint: Keep the client's education materials in a special "Home Care Corner" so all members of the team and the family can have easy access to them.

One of the important skills the nurse uses in home health nursing is teaching and training the client and family. Medicare and other payors of the client's care recognize the importance of education and consider it a reasonable expense. The main focuses for the client who has had a stroke and the family is twofold. First, to focus on restoring the client's functional ability to self-care (or that client's highest level of self-care) and second, to prevent another stroke, including making all necessary lifestyle changes. The nurse on the case develops a teaching plan based on:

- the physician's orders
- the client and family role
- the condition of the client

- the number of visits covered
- the nursing care plan and the HCA care plan
- the long-term and short-term client goals
- the expected outcomes

Factors to consider in the success of any client and family education program include:

- the severity of the illness and what areas of the brain are affected
- ages of the learners and if there were previous strokes
- education level of the learners, taking into consideration that the learning level decreases with a stroke and its disabilities
- emotional status of the learners, especially if the client or family is depressed
- **compliance** (following of teaching plan) level of the client and the family who play such an important role
- motivation level of the client and family
- understanding of importance of education, especially in preventing another stroke
- understanding of importance of goals as they apply to each individual client who has had a stroke

compliance how well the client/family responds to the educational process

The HCA's role in the education process of the client who has had a CVA is to:

1. Serve as a role model and set a good example when providing care and performing procedures.
2. Interact and observe the level of knowledge of the client and the family's ability to learn, and communicate this information to the supervisor or nurse both verbally and in the documentation of visit notes.
3. Offer follow-ups to the teaching if appropriate. This means the HCA must understand as much about strokes as the family and the client are expected to learn. The HCA will **reinforce** the information, both verbal and printed, that is given to the client and family by the nurse and the therapists.

Helpful Hint: The HCA should ask the client and the family to share teaching information and materials so he or she can keep informed.

reinforce strengthen or support

Some examples of observations the HCA might document include:

- nutrition, fluid intake, and diet information as taught by the dietitian
- pain and mobility levels of the client
- exercises as taught by the therapist or nurse and done by the client with the assistance of the HCA or the family
- speech and occupational exercises taught by the therapists, and document the changes and progress seen

- the improvement or deterioration of the client's level of self-care from visit to visit

Situations where the HCA would serve as a role model include:

- motivating the client and the family
- following the HCA care plan
- utilizing infection control practices
- offering a positive and encouraging manner
- practicing good personal hygiene
- displaying a patient and caring attitude (Figure 8-1)
- using proper techniques while performing personal care
- performing procedures well
- following good safety rules
- showing respect for the client's home
- being dependable and courteous

Some situations in which the HCA will have opportunities to interact and observe the client and family's abilities and level of learning include:

- client's verbal communication during ADLs
- family's verbal communication during visit
- client's nonverbal communication behavior during personal care
- family's nonverbal communication behavior during visit
- both family and client when reviewing the care plan

When educating the client who has had a stroke and his or her family, it is important to remember:

1. The environment should be comfortable and quiet with no distractions such as television, radio, or visitors. The attention span of the client who has had a stroke will be shorter than that of other clients.

2. The educational materials should be interesting and at the learner's level of understanding. The materials must take into consideration any disabilities the client may have in learning.

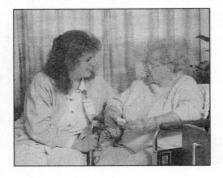

Figure 8–1 The HCA should talk with the client to ensure that he or she understands all the material presented.

3. The teacher should speak slowly and clearly and demonstrate patience by repeating when necessary. If there is a loss of speech in the client who has had a stroke, the teacher should expect only short, simple, verbal responses or gestures.
4. Positive reinforcement, such as praise and not criticism, encourages learning.
5. The educational period should be short, organized, and convenient to the learner. The client responds best to teaching times early in the day before fatigue becomes a factor.
6. The educational content should be taught in a step-by-step plan. The teaching materials should be printed for these cases.
7. The teacher should demonstrate by example and not rush. The education of this client is very slow at first and requires repetition.

empower to authorize or strongly encourage another person

The final result of good client and family education is to **empower** these persons to reach their highest potential. The areas most often addressed in home health care in education are:

- ambulation and exercise, with or without assistive devices
- self-care, such as bathing, skin care, hair and nail care, and mouth care
- elimination from the urinary tract and bowel
- diet and fluid changes
- self-administration of medications
- understanding disease condition risk factors and preventing another stroke
- safety measures, and prevention and treatment of contractures and deformities
- infection control practices
- care and use of physical therapy equipment and assistive devices
- nutrition, diet, preparation of food, and self-feeding
- speech and motor skills
- support groups and additional information

Some specific CVA prevention teaching includes:

- stop smoking
- maintain the ideal weight for a person's height
- check nonprescription drugs with the physician prior to taking
- use a medical identification bracelet that lists a history of stroke
- keep cholesterol down
- wear sturdy shoes
- do not take risks in ambulation

SUMMARY

Because the clients will be affected by the CVA the rest of their lives, their education and that of their families is an important part of the home care plan. The HCA will be asked many questions, and should have a knowledge base that covers the information the client/family are taught. Education in all areas is a continual and never-ending process, especially where an illness is concerned. The HCA should look over the education plan left by the nurse in the home, and be prepared to reinforce the information in an intelligent manner. When questions arise that the HCA cannot answer, it is his or her responsibility to forward the questions to the nurse or supervisor so the answer is presented to the client promptly.

CASE STUDY

Your client is well into the rehabilitation phase of her recovery. The nurse has been visiting three times a day to educate the client and family on the importance of compliance with the medications and reducing risk factors of another CVA. What is your role at this point?

REVIEW QUESTIONS

1. Give examples of the four main goals of client and family education for the client who has had a stroke.

    a. An example of documentation that reflects the client's condition is using _____.

    b. Some observable and reportable family problems might be _____ nutrition.

    c. An example of teaching a therapist or nurse might include that the HCA should reinforce is _____.

    d. An example of the HCA as a role model might be a _____ attitude.

2. List four factors that affect the success of the teaching plan for the client who has had a stroke.

    a.

    b.

    c.

    d.

3. Name two situations in which the HCA can interact with the family and observe the levels of learning.

   a.

   b.

4. Which of the following is *not* one of the factors on which a teaching plan is based?

   a. the long-term and short-term client goals

   b. the physician's orders

   c. the condition of the client

   d. the desires of the family

5. In which of the following situations would the HCA *not* be a role model for the client and family?

   a. practicing good personal hygiene

   b. utilizing good infection control practices

   c. documenting all levels of client care

   d. displaying a patient and caring attitude

6. True or False? The comfort of the environment is important in the learning process by the client and family.

7. True or False? The nurse or therapist will teach infection control measures, but the HCA will serve as a good or bad example.

8. True or False? Every client who has had a CVA is an individual and the teaching plan should reflect this.

9. True or False? The HCA has no part to play in the teaching process.

10. Unscramble the following key term from the chapter: ratvoimot _____

CHAPTER 9

Safety and Emergencies

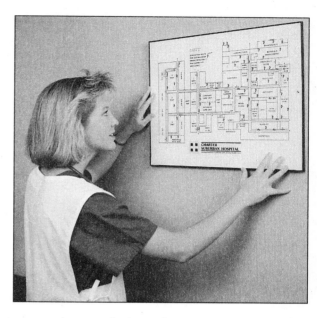

OBJECTIVES

Upon reading this chapter and completing the review questions, the home care aide should be able to:

1. Describe safety and emergency situations in general.
2. Determine the safety level of the environment of the client who has had a stroke.
3. State the most common safety hazards in the home for all clients, focusing on the client who has had a stroke.
4. List some conditions that promote safety and prevent falls.
5. State some basic facts of medication safety.
6. Recognize emergency measures in home care.
7. Demonstrate an understanding of positioning the client and transfer safety.
8. Apply safety measures to the home environment of the client who has had a stroke.

KEY TERMS

anticoagulants
aseptic
confused
disoriented
flammable

pathogens
personal protective equipment (PPE)
safe environment
standard precautions

INTRODUCTION

safe environment an environment in which a person has a very low risk of illness or injury

The home can be an unsafe area for the homebound client as well as for the HCA who cares for that client. Clients who are ill and weak are more prone to accidents at home and are usually unable to handle an emergency. The client who has had a stroke is especially at risk for falls due to the weakness of limbs on one side of the body and the client's use of assistive devices.

Safety is one of the HCA's responsibilities. He or she can create a **safe environment** for the client who has had a stroke by preventing, correcting, or eliminating conditions that could cause accidents and by assisting the client and family in taking measures to be prepared for crisis intervention.

MAINTAINING A SAFE ENVIRONMENT IN THE HOME

When the client who has had a stroke is admitted to home health care, the skilled nurse does a safety assessment of the home during the admission process. A safety checklist is usually included in the admission packet as safety measures and interventions begin at that time. The nurse includes the client's family and the rest of the health care team when setting safety goals and determining if the goals have been met. The HCA follows up on this process. The HCA should constantly assess the quality of the environment and look for safety hazards, and if any are discovered, the HCA should be sure to report them to the supervisor immediately.

A safe environment is one in which a person has a very low risk of illness or injury. Some elderly and frail persons cannot assume the responsibility for their own safety. Poor vision plays a part in a client's inability to be safe at home by leading to falls, tripping, and misreading labels. Hearing loss is another factor affecting the client's safety as warning signals, such as fire detectors, may not be heard.

The assessment of the home environment of the client who has had a stroke should take into consideration this person's disabilities from the stroke. If there is a remaining weakness on one side, the home should be set up to accommodate the weak side. If assistive devices, such as a walker, are to be used, adequate space is needed for the client to move around. Chairs should be sturdy, and not move when sat in, accessible with the walker, and easy to approach. Hallway areas in which the client will walk must have extra wide walking space and be free of extra clutter and rugs. Kitchens should not have tables and chairs that protrude into the walking area which could trip the client. Cabinets should be stocked to permit the client to reach items that are most often used. Sometimes this means leaving items, such as paper towels or dishwashing soaps, out on the counter for easier access.

Helpful Hint: The agency is responsible for the client's safety. Therefore, the HCA as the agency's representative, is also responsible for the client's safety.

flammable   able to catch fire

In bathrooms and bedrooms, the walking areas must be adequate to prevent falls. Drawers and surfaces should be customized so the client can reach all items for self-care.

The most common safety hazards in the home include:

- damaged electrical wiring on large and small appliances
- faulty or uneven stairs
- loose rugs that slip
- poisons
- **flammable** cleaning rags, mops, and brooms
- sharp objects, such as knives, razors, and lawn tools
- wet floors
- cluttered hallways or stairs (Figure 9–1)
- unstable furniture
- electrical cords that are faulty, or too many cords plugged into one outlet (Figure 9–2)

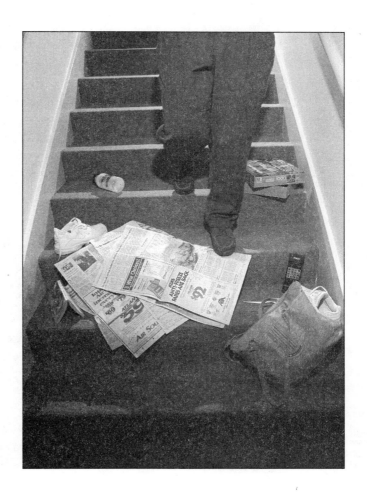

Figure 9–1 A cluttered stairway can be hazardous for the elderly client who has vision or balance problems.

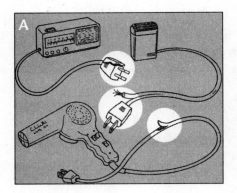 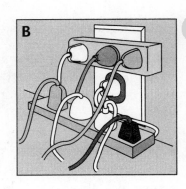

Figure 9–2 A. Cords in unsafe conditions. B. There are too many cords in this outlet.

Falls

Falls are the most common accidents in the home, particularly among the elderly. Most falls occur in the bedroom or bathroom and are caused by slippery floors, throw rugs, poor lighting, cluttered floors, furniture that is out of place, or slippery bathtubs and showers. Some conditions that promote safety and prevent falls are:

- adequate lighting in rooms and hallways.
- hand rails on both sides of stairs, in halls, and in bathrooms (Figure 9–3)

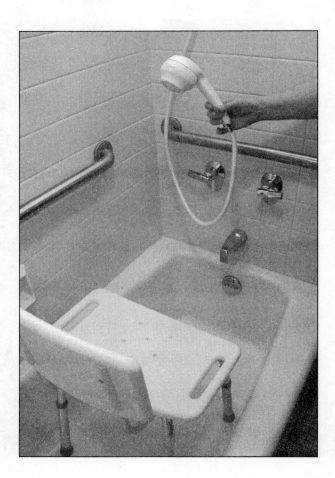

Figure 9–3 Safety features for the tub include several types of bars, nonskid strips, and bathing chair.

- carpeting tacked down and throw rugs avoided
- nonskid shoes and slippers worn by clients when ambulating
- nonskid waxes used on hardwood, tiled, or linoleum floors
- floors uncluttered with toys and other objects
- electrical cords and extension cords kept out of the path of the client
- furniture left in place and not rearranged
- a telephone and lamp placed at the bedside
- nonskid bathmats in tubs and showers
- weak clients assisted to walk, get out of bed, get out of the tub or shower, and with other activities as ordered by the physician
- a call bell within easy reach
- cracked steps, loose hand rails, and frayed carpets reported and repaired promptly
- frequently used items placed within the client's easy reach
- client's bed in the low position except when bedside care is being given to minimize the distance from the bed to the floor if the client falls or gets out of bed
- night lights in the client's room and hallways at night
- floors kept free of spills and excess furniture
- crutches, canes, and walkers fitted with nonskid tips
- wheels on beds and wheelchairs locked when transferring clients to or from them
- gates at the tops and bottoms of stairs when there are infants and toddlers in the home (the child should not be able to put his or her head through the gate bars)
- side rails installed on the client's bed to prevent the client from falling out of bed

Medication Safety

Storage and disposal of medications in the home are major problem areas for home health workers. HCAs should never dispense or administer medication. However, the HCA needs information about certain medications because many clients receiving home care services take them. HCAs often hand medications to their clients, remind clients to take medications, and report their use, misuse, and effects to their supervisors. The client who has had a stroke may be on **anticoagulant** medications to keep the blood thin and free from clots that may cause another stroke. HCAs should know as much about the client's medications as the nurse expects the client and family to know. In the case of anticoagulants, the following are important safety measures:

anticoagulant a medication that prevents or inhibits the clotting of blood

- keep track of the amount of medication left so as not to run out
- always follow the label instructions
- never take aspirin or aspirin products with prescription anticoagulants unless the physician orders it
- bruising occurs easily so avoid bumping and scraping the body
- call the physician for signs of bleeding in stool or urine
- watch for bleeding gums
- crush medications if the client has difficulty swallowing
- if on aspirin for anticoagulation therapy, note signs of bleeding, and have the client drink plenty of fluids, take the aspirin with food, and avoid alcohol.

> **Helpful Hint:** Keep your eyes and ears open for over-the-counter medication use and misuse that should be reported to the nurse and/or supervisor.

The following are some safety guidelines for medications.

1. When cleaning the medicine cabinet, special care should be taken not to disturb medication container labels.
2. Medication containers should be replaced in the same position in the medicine cabinet after cleaning, because clients often expect a bottle to be in one position and do not look at the label.
3. If more than one person in the household is taking medications, keep the medications in separate rooms to avoid a client taking the wrong medication.
4. Encourage the client to dispose of old medications correctly by flushing them down the toilet, and report the disposal to the supervisor.
5. The client should store medications in a specific area and tell the family members where it is; the medications should not be moved.
6. Know if there are special instructions for storage of medications such as refrigeration.
7. Never refer to medications as *candy*.

The *five rights* for safely taking medications are:

1. The *right* client
2. The *right* medication
3. The *right* time
4. The *right* way to take the medication (oral, for example)
5. The *right* dose

EMERGENCY MEASURES IN HOME CARE

> **Helpful Hint:** All HCAs should keep current in CPR and emergency measures at all times.

HCAs may be called upon to handle emergency situations in the home. All HCAs should have a basic first aid course and a current basic life support course.

Emergency Plans

Each emergency situation is different. The following rules apply to any kind of emergency.

1. HCAs should know their limitations and not try a procedure that is unfamiliar.

2. HCAs should remain calm at all times. Being calm helps the victim feel more secure.

3. HCAs should observe the client for life-threatening problems and always check breathing, pulse, and bleeding.

4. HCAs should keep the victim lying down or in the position in which he or she was found; do not move the victim. Moving a victim could make the injury worse.

5. HCAs should perform necessary emergency measures.

6. HCAs should call for help or instruct someone to call 911. An operator will send emergency vehicles and personnel to the scene. The person calling 911 should give the following information to the operator:

   - the location, including the street address and city or town
   - the phone number where the victim is
   - what happened (a fall, for example) since fire equipment, police, and ambulances may be needed
   - how many people require emergency medical attention
   - the conditions of the victims, any obvious injuries, and if there is a life-threatening situation
   - what aid is currently being given

7. HCAs should not remove the victim's clothing unless absolutely necessary.

8. The victim should be kept warm. Aides can cover the victim with a blanket or a coat.

9. HCAs should reassure the conscious victim by explaining what is happening and that help has been called and is on the way.

10. HCAs should not give the victim any foods or fluids.

11. HCAs should keep onlookers away from the victim to maintain his or her privacy.

Every home should have a plan in case of emergencies (Figure 9–4). However, the home with an elderly, frail, ill, or impaired person must take extra measures to plan ahead for emergency situations.

Reporting an accident or emergency by phone should be done in a calm manner. It is important to have emergency phone numbers written next to the telephone (Figure 9–5). This list should include:

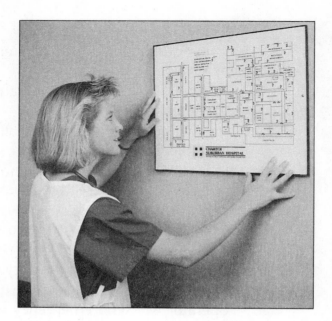

Figure 9–4 Client and family should know the escape plan in the event of a fire.

- Emergency Medical Service (often 911) if available
- police department
- fire department
- responsible family member at work
- the home care supervisor and agency
- client's physician
- nearest hospital
- ambulance service (if other than EMS)
- poison control center

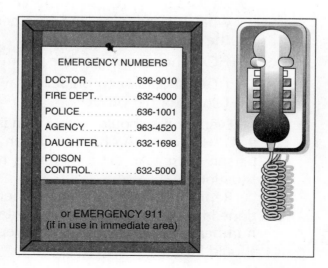

Figure 9–5 Important numbers should be posted by the telephone.

If there is no phone in the client's home, arrange in advance to use a neighbor's phone in case of an emergency.

Emergency care for a possible stroke victim is taught in the American Red Cross first aid course. The four signs of a stroke should be recognized immediately:

1. Weakness or paralysis of one side of the body including:
    - drooping eyelid or mouth
    - affected arms, fingers, legs, and toes
    - poor grasping ability
2. Slurred speech.
3. Staggering walk.
4. Change or loss of consciousness.

    The emergency response is to:
- call for help
- if unconscious, place victim on the affected side to prevent aspiration
- if conscious, raise head and shoulders (except in cases where an unstable neck is suspected; for example, after a fall)
- reassure victims, even if unconscious
- keep body temperature normal
- stay with victims
- do not give food or drink
- get to hospital as soon as possible for treatment

Fire Safety

There are three major causes of fires in this country: faulty electrical equipment and wiring, overloaded electrical circuits, and smoking. In addition if three elements are present in the right proportions, a fire will result (Figure 9–6). The three elements are heat, fuel, and oxygen.

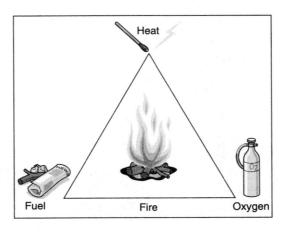

Figure 9–6   The fire triangle—elements needed for combustion (burning)

1. Follow the fire safety precautions for the use of oxygen.
2. Be sure all ashes and cigar and cigarette butts are out before emptying ashtrays.
3. Provide ashtrays to clients who are allowed to smoke.
4. Empty ashtrays into a metal container partly filled with sand or water. Do not empty ashtrays into wastebaskets or plastic containers lined with paper or plastic bags.
5. Supervise the smoking of clients who cannot protect themselves. This includes **confused**, **disoriented**, and sedated clients.
6. Follow the safety practices for using electrical equipment.
7. Supervise the play of children and keep matches out of their reach.

confused uncertain or unclear mentally

disoriented confusion in the sense of identity or location

The following guidelines will help the HCA to protect the client if there is a fire. The HCA should:

1. Call the fire department (have fire emergency numbers near the client's phones).
2. Plan escape routes from each room.
3. Know where fire extinguishers are located and how to use them.
4. Know where fire alarm boxes are located.
5. Turn off any oxygen or electrical equipment in the general area of the fire.
6. Get the client and others out of the house.
7. Try to fight a small fire if you can. Leave right away if the fire gets out of control.
8. Close door if the home is vacated.
9. Crawl, keeping the client's head close to the floor if the area is filled with smoke.
10. Cover the client's face with a damp cloth or towel if in a smoke-filled area (Figure 9–7).
11. Feel any doors before they are opened. Do not open a door that feels hot or if smoke is coming from around the door.
12. When opening a cool door, open slowly, keeping the head to the side. Doors should be closed immediately if smoke or heat rushes in.
13. Stuff blankets, clothes, towels, linens, coats, or other cloth at the bottom of the door if the client is trapped inside. A window should be opened for air and a piece of cloth hung outside the window to attract attention.

The HCA should be able to use a fire extinguisher (Figure 9–8A and B). Local fire departments often give demonstrations on how to operate a fire extinguisher and some agencies require all employees to demonstrate how to use them.

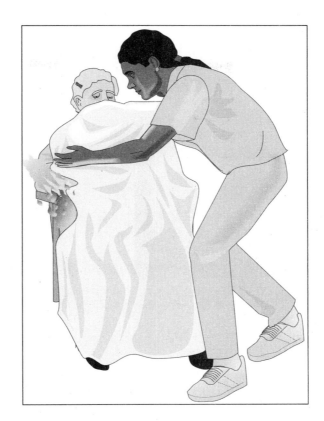

Figure 9–7 The HCA protects the client while trying to extinguish the fire.

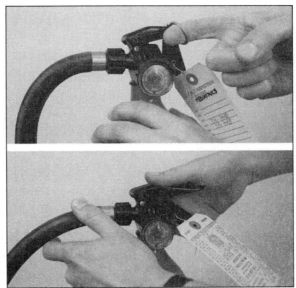

Figure 9–8 To use a fire extinguisher, (A) remove pin and (B) push top handle down.

> **Helpful Hint:** The HCA should remember that the escape of a disabled client will be slower than others.

The RACE system is used as a general guideline in fire safety (Figure 9–9).

- **R**emove the client from immediate danger
- **A**ctivate the alarm (or call the fire department) to alert others
- **C**onfine the fire by closing doors
- **E**xtinguish the fire, if possible

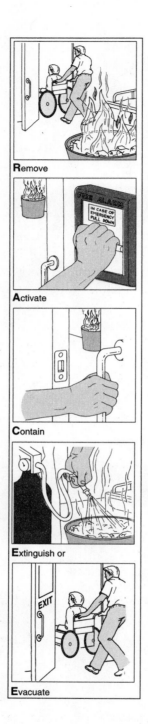

Remove

Activate

Contain

Extinguish or

Evacuate

Figure 9–9   R-A-C-E Procedure

INFECTION CONTROL

All home health personnel must be careful to use proper measures to control infection. The client who has had a stroke is at no greater or lesser risk for infection than any other client. Specialized HCAs should keep current on the latest information to protect the client, family, other workers, and themselves from infection. The Centers for Disease Control (CDC) published new recommendations in 1996 for standard precautions. This new information is founded on several years of research and data collection to:

- improve the criteria for universal precautions
- change some of the medical terminology
- offer new information on drug resistant pathogens
- update isolation guidelines

Standard Precautions

standard precautions new guidelines which replace the original universal precautions of infection control

Universal precautions were developed in 1985 by the CDC. These guidelines were adhered to until they were updated in 1996 to **standard precautions** (Figure 9–10). These new guidelines apply to all health care workers on all clients, no matter what their diagnosis or where they are being cared for. If proper precautions are not taken, pathogens can be transmitted by the HCAs to themselves, their families, other clients, and their families by way of skin and clothing. Standard precautions protect against many different types of infections including AIDS, tuberculosis (TB), and Hepatitis B (HBV).

Personal Protective Equipment (PPE)

personal protective equipment (PPE) devices such as masks, gowns, gloves, and face shields which form a barrier between you and an infectious environment

Personal Protective Equipment provides a barrier between the client and health care worker. When used correctly, PPE provides a barrier that prevents the transfer of pathogens from one person to another. Standard precautions require all health care workers to wear PPE anytime they expect to have contact with

- blood
- any moist body fluid except sweat, secretions, or excretions
- mucous membranes
- nonintact skin

PPE includes gloves, water-resistant gowns, face shields or masks, and goggles. HCAs should follow their agency's policies for use of PPE in routine tasks.

Some new medical terms associated with infection control include:

Visible—able to be seen with the eye

Body Substance Isolation—precautions requiring special handling of all fluids

Drug Resistant—disease-causing organisms that resist treatment with normal antibiotics

Reservoir—a human being who has an infection that can be spread to others

Airborne Transmission—tiny microbes spread in the air over long distances, such as TB

STANDARD PRECAUTIONS FOR INFECTION CONTROL

Wash Hands (Plain soap)
Wash after touching blood, body fluids, secretions, excretions, and contaminated items. Wash immediately after gloves are removed and between patient contacts. Avoid transfer of microorganisms to other patients or environments.

Wear Gloves
Wear when touching blood, body fluids, secretions, excretions, and contaminated items. Put on clean gloves just before touching mucous membranes and nonintact skin. Change gloves between tasks and procedures on the same patient after contact with material that may contain high concentrations of microorganisms. Remove gloves promptly after use, before touching noncontaminated items and environmental surfaces, and before going to another patient, and wash hands immediately to avoid transfer of microorganisms to other patients or environments.

Wear Mask and Eye Protection or Face Shield
Protect mucous membranes of the eyes, nose and mouth during procedures and patient-care activities that are likely to generate splashes or sprays of blood, body fluids, secretions, or excretions.

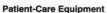

Wear Gown
Protect skin and prevent soiling of clothing during procedures that are likely to generate splashes or sprays of blood, body fluids, secretions, or excretions. Remove a soiled gown as promptly as possible and wash hands to avoid transfer of microorganisms to other patients or environments.

Patient-Care Equipment
Handle used patient-care equipment soiled with blood, body fluids, secretions, or excretions in a manner that prevents skin and mucous membrane exposures, contamination of clothing, and transfer of microorganisms to other patients and environments. Ensure that reusable equipment is not used for the care of another patient until it has been appropriately cleaned and reprocessed and single use items are properly discarded.

Environmental Control
Follow hospital procedures for routine care, cleaning, and disinfection of environmental surfaces, beds, bedrails, bedside equipment and other frequently touched surfaces.

Linen
Handle, transport, and process used linen soiled with blood, body fluids, secretions, or excretions in a manner that prevents exposure and contamination of clothing, and avoids transfer of microorganisms to other patients and environments.

Occupational Health and Bloodborne Pathogens
Prevent injuries when using needles, scalpels, and other sharp instruments or devices; when handling sharp instruments after procedures; when cleaning used instruments; and when disposing of used needles.

Never recap used needles using both hands or any other technique that involves directing the point of a needle towards any part of the body; rather, use either a one-handed "scoop" technique or a mechanical device designed for holding the needle sheath.

Do not remove used needles from disposable syringes by hand, and do not bend, break, or otherwise manipulate used needles by hand. Place used disposable syringes and needles, scalpels, blades, and other sharp items in puncture-resistant sharps containers located as close as practical to the area in which the items were used, and place reusable syringes and needles in a puncture-resistant container for transport to the reprocessing area.

Use resuscitation devices as an alternative to mouth-to-mouth resuscitation.

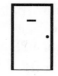

Patient Placement
Use a private room for a patient who contaminates the environment or who does not (or cannot be expected to) assist in maintaining appropriate hygiene or environmental control. Consult Infection Control if a private room is not available.

Figure 9–10   Standard precautions (Courtesy of BREVIS Corporation, Salt Lake City, UT).

Droplet Transmission—disease spread by respiratory secretions or droplets in the air within a distance of three feet

Transmission-Based Precautions—CDC recommendations for isolating clients with certain diseases, in addition to standard precautions

Higher-Efficiency Particulate Air Mask (HEPA)—a special mask with tiny pores to prevent airborne transmissions

Table 9–1 lists some of the diseases requiring transmission-based precautions.

Pathogens, which are the cause of infections, can be controlled with good cleaning techniques and maintenance. It is important to keep an **aseptic** environment for the client. Some common aseptic practices include:

• washing hands before and after touching the client

pathogens disease-causing microorganisms

aseptic free of disease-causing pathogens

Table 9–1 Diseases Requiring Transmission-Based Isolation Precautions	
Disease or Condition	**Type of Precautions**
AIDS	Standard (or reverse if facility policy)
Chicken pox	Airborne and Contact
Diarrhea	Standard
Drug-resistant skin infections	Contact
German measles	Droplet
Head or body lice	Contact
Hepatitis, type A	Standard. Use contact if diarrhea or incontinent patient
Hepatitis, other types	Standard
HIV disease	Standard
Impetigo	Contact
Infected pressure sore with no drainage	Standard
Infected pressure sore with heavy drainage	Contact
Infectious diarrhea caused by a known pathogen	Contact
Measles	Airborne
Mumps	Droplet
Oral or genital herpes	Standard
Scabies	Contact
Syphilis	Standard
Tuberculosis of the lungs	Airborne
Widespread shingles	Airborne and Contact
Use standard precautions in addition to other types of precautions listed.	

- washing hands after urinating, having a bowel movement, or changing tampons or sanitary napkins
- washing hands before handling or preparing food
- washing fruits and vegetables before serving them
- encouraging each family member to use his or her own towels, washcloths, toothbrush, drinking glass, and other personal care items
- using disposable cups and dishes for clients with an infection
- encouraging the client to cover the nose and mouth with tissues when coughing, sneezing, or blowing the nose.
- making sure there is a plastic or paper bag for used tissues
- practicing good personal hygiene by bathing, washing hair, and brushing teeth regularly
- encouraging clients to wash their hands often, especially after toileting and before eating
- washing cooking and eating utensils with soap and water after they have been used
- cleaning cooking and eating surfaces with soap and water or a disinfectant

- not leaving food sitting out and uncovered; closing all food containers; refrigerating foods that will spoil
- not using food that smells bad or looks discolored
- checking the expiration date on food and not using it if the date has passed
- changing water in flower vases daily
- removing dead plants and flowers from the home
- dusting furniture with a damp cloth and using a damp mop for floors to help prevent the movement of dust in the air
- emptying garbage every day using large, sturdy plastic bags or wrapping the garbage in several thicknesses of newspaper.
- placing the garbage outside the home in plastic or metal garbage containers
- wearing disposable gloves if there are open cuts or sores on hands
- holding equipment and linens away from uniform
- not shaking linens to prevent the movement of dust
- cleaning from the cleanest area to the dirtiest to prevent soiling a clean area
- cleaning away from the body and uniform because wiping toward oneself transmits microorganisms to the skin, hair, and uniform
- pouring contaminated liquids directly into sinks or toilets and avoiding splashes of liquid onto other areas
- not sitting on the client's bed if the client has an infection to prevent picking up microorganisms and carrying them to the next surface
- wearing disposable gloves during contact with the client's body fluids, such as when giving enemas, cleaning the client's genital area, handling vomitus, or giving mouth care.
- wearing a disposable apron when in contact with the client's body fluids

SUMMARY

Promoting a safe and healthy environment for the client rests in the hands of the HCA. There are certain standards and practices that must be maintained when the client is under the care of the agency. These include the prevention of accidents as well as infection control practices that meet the Occupational Safety and Health Administration's (OSHA) state and local regulations. Emergency situations sometimes occur and HCAs are expected to respond to them in a professional manner that puts the safety of the client first.

CASE STUDY

If your client has a right-side hemiplegia, what special considerations would be important in making the environment at home safe? Include the possibility of an emergency in your answer.

REVIEW QUESTIONS

1. A safe environment is defined as:

2. List two sensory disabilities that affect the elderly clients safety.
    a.

    b.

3. List the five precautions when taking anticoagulation medications.
    a.

    b.

    c.

    d.

    e.

4. Who does the admission safety assessment of the client and the home?

    a. physician

    b. risk manager

    c. nurse

    d. HCA

5. Which of the following are common safety hazards for a client who has had a stroke?

    a. spills on floors

    b. damaged wiring

    c. poisons left unlabeled

    d. cluttered hallways

    e. all of the above

6. Which of the following is *not* an HCA responsibility?

    a. safe storage of medications

    b. administering medications

    c. assisting the client with medications

    d. measuring medications

7. True or False? If more than one person in a household is taking medication, the medications should be placed in separate rooms.

8. True or False? Old medications should not be flushed down the toilet.

9. True or False? The HCA should get the possible stroke victim to the hospital quickly in emergency situations.

10. True or False? It is never acceptable to cover the client's face with a damp cloth when escaping a smoke-filled room.

11. True or False? The CDC has developed new universal precautions entitled standard precautions.

12. True or False? The HCA can lower the risk of transmission of pathogens by using proper hand-washing procedures.

13. Unscramble the following key term from the chapter: ltagcnioutnaa _____

Abuse

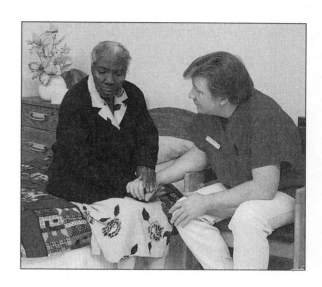

OBJECTIVES

Upon reading this chapter and completing the review questions, the home care aide should be able to:

1. Define abuse.
2. Identify six types of abuse and/or neglect.
3. Identify factors contributing to adult abuse.
4. Identify physical indicators of adult abuse, neglect, and exploitation.
5. State the client's rights.

KEY TERMS

abuse	retaliation
exploitation	self-abuse
intervention	self-respect
negligence	standard of practice
respect	

INTRODUCTION

Many elderly persons live rich and productive lives with positive relationships with their children and friends. On the other hand, many are severely disabled, living in institutions, and twice that number live with and are dependent on their children or siblings. Those elderly persons who are dependent are often a physical, financial, and emotional strain on those persons and families who care for them. Caring for a dependent older adult in the home can cost up to twenty-five thousand dollars a year. Custodial care is not a Medicare reimbursable service and is rarely covered by other health insurance policies. With these factors common in our society, the 1990s have seen an increase in the neglect and abuse of the elderly population. The client who is left with permanent disabilities after a stroke is at a high risk for abuse because of mental and physical limitations leading to a dependency on others for assistance. Even those clients whose rehabilitation is excellent will have some lifestyle changes that may make him or her more at risk for abuse.

abuse is defined as the infliction of physical pain or injury or any persistent course of conduct intended to produce or result in mental or emotional distress. Severe neglect and severe physical abuse cause great distress and pain and can lead to injury or death. Figure 10–1 shows a client who may have been abused.

Clients who have had a CVA are not fully able to care for themselves and are an easy target for abuse. This abuse can be administered by untrained, frustrated, or overburdened family members or by those who deliberately harm others for their own gain.

abuse inflicting physical or mental pain or injury on another person

SIX TYPES OF ABUSE

HCAs are in a position to notice signs of abuse or neglect. If either is occurring, whatever is seen should be handled confidentially. Any signs or suspicions of abuse should be immediately reported to the supervisor.

There are six types of abuse or neglect to watch out for:

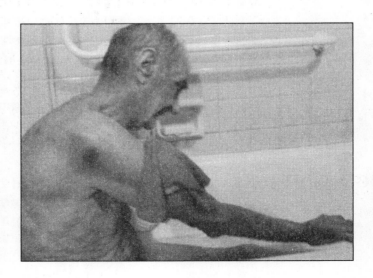

Figure 10–1 Note the bruise on the client's shoulder. The HCA should observe the client, and report any possible signs of abuse to the supervisor.

1. Passive Neglect—Harm is not intended, but occurs because some type of care is not being provided because of the caregiver's inability, laziness, or lack of knowledge.

2. Psychological Abuse—Harm caused to the client's feelings or emotional state by demeaning, frightening, humiliating, intimidating, isolating, insulting him or her, treating the client as a child, or by using verbal aggression.

3. Material or Financial Abuse—Stealing, **exploitation**, or improperly using the money, property, or other assets of the elderly client.

4. Active Neglect—Intentionally harming the older person physically or psychologically by failing to provide needed care. Examples include deliberately leaving a bedridden person alone for lengthy periods or willfully denying the person food, medication, dentures, or eyeglasses.

5. Physical Abuse—Intentionally harming the person physically by slapping, bruising, sexually molesting, cutting, burning, physically restraining, pushing, or shoving.

6. **Self-Abuse** or Self-Neglect—Any of the five activities mentioned above committed by the older person against himself or herself.

The key is for the HCA to be alert to the physical and mental condition of the client at all times, and to report changes and unusual conditions to the supervisor regularly and promptly.

exploitation   to use selfishly or unethically

self-abuse   refusal to care for oneself

REPORTING ABUSE

Your supervisor must be informed of any suspicions you may have in order to help identify the proper action to take regarding the abusive behavior. In order to protect the victim, the situation must be handled carefully; the supervisor and other professionals will become involved if it appears that abuse is taking place. Because the client who has had a CVA may already feel a burden to the family, he or she will tolerate destructive behavior from caregivers more than will other types of clients. These clients who are in a more weakened condition do not feel they have a right to complain about unacceptable behaviors from caregivers. Loss of thinking ability makes it more difficult for him or her to understand what possible options there could be for changing a situation involving abuse. This hopelessness is often associated with feelings of loss of control over one's life, especially when one is no longer able to work and earn a living. Home health personnel may be the only influences for motivating these persons to change their lives.

Helpful Hint: According to the law, domestic violence and elderly or child abuse must be reported by health caregivers.

The primary reasons for not reporting elderly abuse are:

- fear of personal involvement
- lack of evidence that abuse has occurred
- lack of response by authorities
- a generalized belief that reported cases are not satisfactorily handled

There is a legal responsibility of health care providers to report discovered cases of abuse, neglect, or exploitation. Forty-one states have laws that mandate the reporting of elder abuse. The law usually states that health professionals or persons who have knowledge of, or who reasonably suspect, abuse must report it. The states also protect the health personnel from civil or criminal liability for the content of the report. Each state has its own laws, and penalties are issued in some states for not reporting abuse.

FACTORS CONTRIBUTING TO ELDERLY ABUSE

The factors contributing to adult abuse include

retaliation repayment in kind; usually revenge

- **retaliation**
- ageism and violence as a way of life
- lack of close family ties
- lack of community resources
- lack of financial resources
- mental and emotional disorders
- unemployment
- history of alcohol and drug abuse
- environmental conditions
- resentment of dependency
- increased life expectancy
- other situational stresses

Many of these factors apply to the family situation of the client who is weakened by a stroke.

SIGNS OF ELDERLY ABUSE

The three main indicators of adult abuse are:

1. Personal factors, such as ignorance and emotional disturbance.
2. Interpersonal factors, such as unresolved conflicts and lack of gratitude.
3. Situational factors, such as the dependent person living with his or her children and their families, thus causing feelings of frustration and stress to the caregiver.

Physical signs of adult (elderly) abuse, neglect, or exploitation are:

- unexplained bruises or welts
- unexplained fractures
- unexplained burns
- unexplained lacerations or abrasions
- mental confusion
- poor personal hygiene
- denial of pain when pain is obvious
- bedbound but not related to the disease
- weight loss
- dehydration
- old, unexplained scars
- fearfulness and noncommunicative

Some behavioral signs of abuse are evident when the client:

- yells obscenities at others
- threatens self-harm or suicide
- refuses medical care
- shows unrealistic fear or hostility
- shows signs of alcohol or drug abuse
- experiences denial of the situation
- stops communicating
- is fearful to be alone (Figure 10–2A)
- cries excessively (Figure 10–2B)
- displays anger at the family
- has a poor self-concept and shows poor self-control
- shows signs of hopelessness

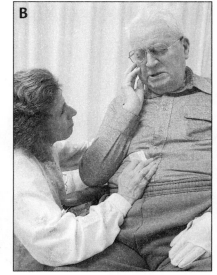

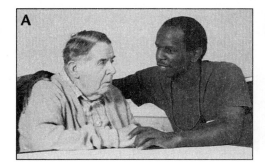

Figure 10–2 Signs of possible behavioral abuse. (A) the client is afraid to be alone. (B) the client experiences excessive crying.

Environmental signs of elderly abuse are evident when:

- the house is dirty and there is garbage around
- there are fleas, mice, and vermin present in the home
- the home is overcrowded
- the home smells of urine or feces
- the home is not kept at a comfortable temperature
- pets are not well cared for
- there are empty bottles of liquor or medicine containers lying around
- the bed sheets are dirty and have not been changed
- there is not enough food in the home
- the food is spoiled and the refrigerator is dirty
- the food is stored improperly
- there are no special foods for the client's diet
- there is no cash available
- there are unusual withdrawals of money at the bank
- the client complains of having no money or that the family is stealing money from the client

negligence lack of care that would usually be expected

standard of practice the policies and procedures which form the basis for providing adequate care to an ill or injured client

Negligence occurs when a health caregiver does not give the care expected by a set **standard of practice** (what the average person with the same training would do). This includes not following established policies and procedures in providing client care. If an HCA fails to put the side rails up on the client's bed and he or she falls during the night, that is considered negligence. Also, if the HCA fails to report a situation of abuse by a family member to a client, the state considers the HCA equally guilty if harm comes to the client.

Some forms of abuse which might be seen in weakened clients after a stroke include:

- humiliation of the client by yelling or teasing
- not changing positions when the client cannot do it himself or herself
- placing the client without his or her permission in a wheelchair or a room
- forcing a client to eat, or not feeding a person who can't feed himself or herself
- making fun of the way a person speaks
- punishing a client who is incontinent by not changing a diaper
- improperly using restraints

SUBSTANCE ABUSE IN THE ELDERLY

Substance abuse is a causative factor in elderly abuse and abuse of alcohol is a major health problem. The third most common mental disorder in elderly men is alcoholism. Some signs the HCA can watch for in clients that may indicate alcoholism are:

- poor personal hygiene
- nutritional problems (weight loss)
- neglect of home
- depression
- suicidal ideas
- repeated falls
- flushed face
- tremors
- extreme fatigue
- incontinence
- withdrawal

HCAs should discuss any suspected substance abuse with the supervisor so that the physician can be notified and orders for **intervention** and referral given. The HCA should communicate well with the client in order to determine if substance abuse is occurring (Figure 10–3).

PREVENTION OF ABUSE

Some suggestions to give to patients to prevent abuse and maintain independence are:

- keep a network of friends and activities as long as possible
- participate in community activities
- have a "buddy system" with a friend outside of the family and communicate weekly
- make and keep personal care appointments such as dentist and hairdresser

intervention any measure which modifies treatment or alters the course of a disease

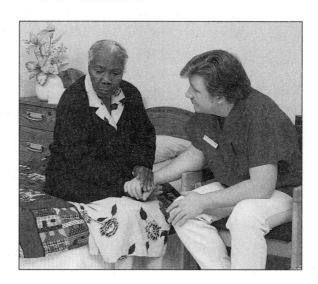

Figure 10–3 The HCA should be especially alert to any possible signs of abuse, and report them to the supervisor immediately.

- invite guests to the home frequently
- maintain your own telephone
- be neat and organized
- do not leave valuables around
- do not give up financial control unless absolutely necessary

RESPECT

respect regard of one person for another

Respect is defined as special regard by one person for another. Respect for clients means being fair and decent toward them at all times. It also means having regard for the client's life and being committed to caring for them to maintain a higher quality of life. Respect for another individual includes seeing that the person's life has value, even when there is a disease or illness present.

Each person is different in a unique and special way. Human beings, when they are ill, such as the client who has had a stroke, are very dependent on others for care. They also look to those caregivers to gain back their **self-respect** which is similar to self-esteem. Self-respect comes from outside oneself and inside oneself. When others respect you, you also respect yourself. But in many ways, respect is based on extremely strong principles and high moral codes of behavior.

self-respect regard of one person for himself or herself

These include:
- obeying laws
- following rules
- not damaging property
- loyalty toward friends and family
- belief in a higher power
- being honest and fair
- accepting human differences

CLIENTS' RIGHTS

The clients' Bill of Rights was developed and published by the American Hospital Association. It has been adopted by home health agencies and has become an important philosophy for all health care workers to learn and apply. Rights are defined as powers or privileges which are appropriate and correct. Recognizing that clients have personal rights is a way of giving them some power and control over their situation. In the case of illness, they often feel they have very little of either.

The rights described in the Bill of Rights include the right to:
- consideration and respect
- current medical information
- information before consent to care

- refuse treatment
- privacy
- confidentiality
- financial information

It is important for HCAs to call all clients by their names. They should always feel secure that their needs and wishes are of the utmost importance to all the staff members.

When the client is in his or her own home, that environment should be respected by the HCA at all times. When client's are admitted for home care, the agency usually provides them with a copy of their rights and responsibilities. Some other rights frequently included are the right to file complaints concerning neglect or abuse with state regulatory authorities. They have the right to voice complaints concerning their care and about staff members. Clients have the right to be free from any form of abuse including verbal abuse.

Clients are informed about their responsibilities while being cared for by an agency. They are responsible for following the physician's medical orders as described on the nurse and HCA care plans. They are also responsible for showing the same respect to the staff that they receive. It is an important client responsibility to be cooperative and agreeable when the HCA is offering care. Respect works when it is a two-way action. The HCA respects the client, the home, and the family. In return, the client must respect the HCA for the training, skills, and care he or she is providing to the client.

Some examples of including client rights in their day-to-day activities are:

1. The HCA calls clients to tell them he or she will be late for the visit
2. The HCA refers questions clients ask about their condition to the supervisor so the nurse or physician can follow up with the answers
3. The HCA reports observed and repeated episodes of verbal abuse toward clients from the family member who is in the home providing care
4. The HCA closes the bedroom or bathroom door when the client is in risk of being exposed.

HCAs should have respect for their clients, the agency, the community, their profession, themselves, and the important role they play in our society. The client responds to the HCA's show of respect by being cooperative and polite.

SUMMARY

No one wants to believe that one person could hurt another, but sometimes abuse does occur, and HCAs are the ones who are exposed to such situations. All humans, but especially persons who are ill and at a disadvantage, have rights to be protected from illegal or unethical actions against them. Clients who are weak and disabled, such as those recovering from a CVA, are especially at risk for abuse. There is a legal and moral responsibility for the HCA to be knowledgeable concerning abuse and to report it when it occurs.

CASE STUDY

You suspect that the aide who sees your client on your days off is using abusive words toward the client and not doing the complete care as ordered by the care plan. What action should you take?

REVIEW QUESTIONS

State the type of abuse described in each of the following situations (Questions 1–5):

1. A daughter helps her elderly mother by cashing, depositing, and managing all of her income. All purchases and household bills were made for the mother by the daughter using her mother's checkbook. The daughter, unfortunately, also paid her own bills from her mother's account. _____

2. A wife cares for her overweight husband at home after a heart attack. A hospital bed was purchased, but the wife was never instructed to turn the patient or give skin care. After turning the husband three months later, she and the neighbor discovered that he had developed three large bedsores. _____

3. A couple cared for the wife's elderly mother in their home. The patient was very confused and constantly caused disruptions, so her bedroom was cleared and she was locked in day and night. The couple insisted they did the best they could. The mother was moved to a nursing home, but the couple refused to pay the bill. _____

4. A daughter asked her elderly mother to move in with her after her divorce. The daughter began to date and was away a lot during the evening. The daughter began to resent the mother's verbal concerns. Excessive name-calling and threats to the mother persisted. The mother ran away for three days and was returned in a frightened state by the police. _____

5. An alcoholic son lived with his elderly, sick, and obese mother in her home. She was hospitalized for fractures of the hip and jaw and bruises on her face and body. The neighbors complained that the son would not allow his mother to leave the house and she died shortly thereafter. Autopsy reports showed regular beatings had taken place. _____

6. Which of the following are possible signs of abuse in the elderly?
   a. no access to bank account
   b. pressure sores
   c. poor hygiene
   d. fearfulness
   e. all of the above
7. Behavioral signs of elderly abuse include:
   a. bruises and welts
   b. crying and depression
   c. fearfulness
   d. burns
8 True or False? HCAs can make a difference in helping the client who has had a stroke to maintain independence.
9. True or False? The HCA is required by law to report suspected abuse.
10. True or False? A sign of potential abuse is that there is garbage left around the home and the family pets are not well cared for.
11. Unscramble the following key word from the chapter: ronntivieent _____

11

Psychosocial Influences

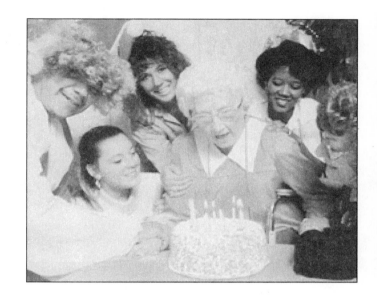

OBJECTIVES

Upon reading this chapter and completing the review questions, the home care aide should be able to:

1. Define psychosocial influences on the client and his or her recovery.
2. Define holistic care of the client who has had a CVA.
3. Explain multicultural differences and human needs.
4. Describe family dynamics and current changes that may affect the client.
5. Be familiar with positive attitudes and codes of behavior for HCAs.
6. Understand disabilities and human responses to them.
7. Understand the communication process, especially with the client who has had a stroke.

KEY TERMS

advocate
confidentiality
cultures
disability

family dynamics
impairments
prognosis
psychosocial

INTRODUCTION

prognosis expected outcome of an illness or injury based on client history, limitations, compliance, and progress

advocate a supporter; one who looks out for the safety and well-being of the client

Most of the clients receiving home health care live in a family-structured environment. The psycho (emotional) social (human interactions) influences on the client may affect the **prognosis** (course of illness). The HCA needs to be aware of these influential factors to better provide the client with a more holistic approach.

THE HOLISTIC CARING MODEL

The holistic caring model is the one which considers the whole client, including mind, body, spiritual well-being, economy, family support, culture, and ethics, not just the illness or disease process, and how these factors can affect the recovery of the client (Figure 11–1).

The HCA serves as a client **advocate** (supporter) but this cannot be successful without an understanding of the uniqueness and variety of types of clients and families with needs that require special care and concern. Figure 11–2 shows an HCA who is concerned about his client.

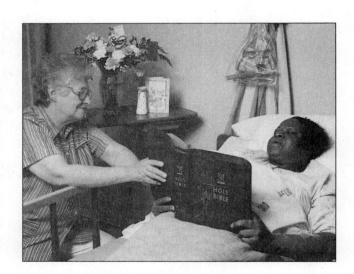

Figure 11–1 Spiritual needs may be greater during illness.

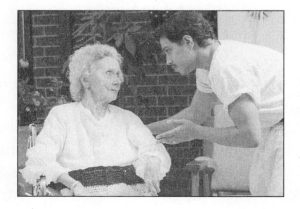

Figure 11–2 The HCA respects differences in clients and families, and understands that each client has needs that require special care and concern.

The United States has a growing population of aging clients as well as an increasing multicultural and multiethnic mix. Figure 11–3 shows six ethnic groups that predominate in the United States. The HCA of the 1990s will be placed in the homes of clients with differences that could effect the level of care or create barriers to the relationship. Some of the barriers the HCA may see in the home are:

- language differences
- discrimination and distrust
- poverty
- resistance to outside help
- culture bias
- negative attitude toward Western health care
- religious practices
- lack of knowledge of medical system
- lack of education
- misunderstood family structure

Multicultural differences may occur in race, religion, language, diet, gender, age, culture, economic status, and lifestyle. Figure 11–4 shows the many ways clients differ. Table 11–1 shows the differences in dietary practices of certain religions.

One area all human beings have in common are their basic needs. A need must be met for a client's well-being. The health caregiver should focus on the client/family's needs first, then

Helpful Hint: If you believe there is a cultural barrier between you and your client or the family, discuss a change of assignment with your supervisor.

Caucasian	England, Scotland, Ireland, Poland, Scandinavia, Italy, Russia	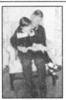	**Asian/Pacific**	China, Japan, Philippines, Vietnam, Cambodia, Korea, Hawaii, Samoa	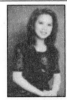
African American	Africa, Haiti, Jamaica, Dominican Republic	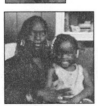	**Native American**	Tribes, such as Cherokee, Apache, Navajo, Blackfoot, Inuit (Alaskan)	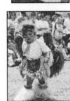
Hispanic	Cuba, Puerto Rico, Mexico, Latin and South America	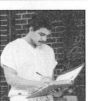	**Middle Eastern**	Egypt, Iran, Yemen, Palestine, Lebanon, Jordan, Saudi Arabia, Kuwait	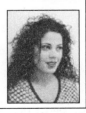

Figure 11–3 Major ethnic groups of America

Table 11–1 Religious Dietary Practices

Faith	Christian Science	Roman Catholic	Muslim Moslem	Seventh Day Adventist	Some Baptists	Greek Orthodox (on fast days)
Restricted Food						
Coffee	•			•	•	
Tea	•			•	•	
Alcohol	•		•	•	•	
Pork/pork products			•	•		
Caffeine-containing foods				•		
Dairy products						•
All meats		1 hour before communion; Ash Wed., Good Friday		Small groups		•

In addition, the Jewish Orthodox faith:
- forbids the serving of milk and milk products with meats
- forbids cooking of food on the Sabbath
- forbids eating of leavened bread during Passover
- observes specific fast days

assess the differences and merge the two to create a care plan for each individual situation. All humans have the following needs:

Daily physical needs:

- food and water
- safety and shelter
- activity and rest
- freedom from pain and discomfort

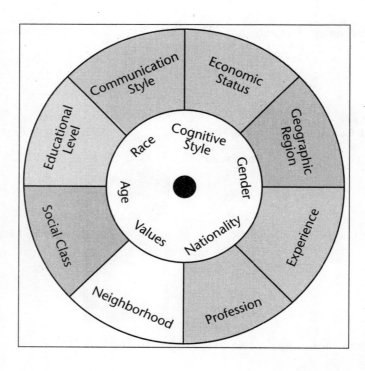

Figure 11–4 Ways in which people differ

Daily psychological needs
- independence and security
- affection and love
- acceptance and social interaction (Figure 11–5)
- trust and dignity
- self-esteem and relationships
- knowledge and achievement

FAMILY DYNAMICS

The family as a unit has changed over the past few decades. The primary family (formerly mother, father, and children) is now frequently made up of step-parents, step-children, and half-brothers and sisters. The extended family (grandparents, aunts, and uncles) who used to live in the same location are now scattered over large geographical areas. As travel became easier, families moved to separate parts of the country. Changes seen in the family unit have been the result of many factors such as:
- smaller families
- single-parent families
- divorces and second marriages
- interracial families
- two-career families
- same-sex households
- aging elderly
- baby boomers
- multicultural families
- diversity and blending of ethnic groups

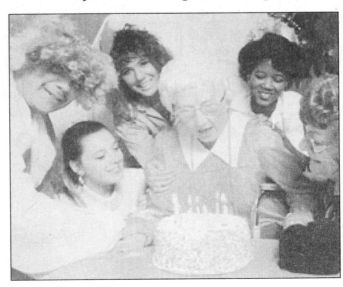

Figure 11–5 Socialization and activities are important components of rehabilitative care.

family dynamics   how the
family interacts

Given all of these factors, the **family dynamics** in the home are also greatly influenced. Other factors contributing to differences in the family that may affect the client who has had a stroke include:

- increase in medical technology
- growth of new minority groups
- blend of cultures in diet, religion, and customs
- differences in health practices and beliefs
- family structure
- language and communication barriers

All of these factors and differences may influence the client and family's behavior. Acceptance by the health care members is the key to understanding these differences. However, if the HCA believes the behavior may in some way interfere with the client's recovery, it is important to report this to the supervisor.

COMMUNICATION

Of all the factors affecting the relationships and interactions between client/family and the HCA, communication is so important it requires further discussion. The United States is a melting pot of many cultures with many different languages and various methods of communication. In addition, the client may be a relatively young person with new **impairments** which can create even more problems in the communication process.

impairments   disabilities caused
by accident or illness

Proper communication is not only what is said but also the way it is expressed, and includes gestures and facial expressions. A positive and cheerful attitude, which is also professional, promotes a trusting relationship between the HCA and the client (Figure 11–6).

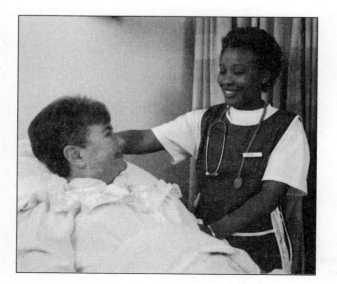

Figure 11–6   A positive and cheerful attitude promotes a trusting relationship between the HCA and the client.

Some general guidelines to improve communication skills include the following:

- attitude should be calm and supportive
- touch and a caring behavior can be effective in reassuring the client (Figure 11–7)
- eye contact should be maintained
- speaking should be slow and distinct with a lower pitch and tone
- only one question should be asked at a time, and plenty of time allowed for responses
- communication should show respect and dignity to the client
- speaking should be slow when conversing with friends and family; each word must be spoken clearly, especially when speaking to someone hard of hearing or to someone whose native language is not English
- HCAs should learn to listen and be patient until the message is completed by the sender, even if the sender has a difficult time stating the message; time spent here is time saved later
- when talking with persons from another culture, HCAs should not try using the words and phrases from different cultures as some of them may have special meanings; if the client and/or family wish to teach special vocabularies and words, setting up an agreed-upon mode of communication can be helpful
- reporting and recording of events should be done in simple terms and sentences

Communicating with the family members may be vital in gaining information important to the nurse and/or physician. However, the HCA must remember that persons who speak

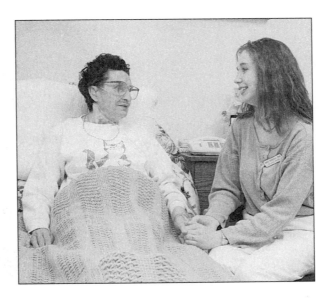

Figure 11–7   Touching residents is important for restorative care.

English as a second language speak more slowly than other clients and must not be rushed. Noise and distractions should be kept to a minimum and short, simple words and sentences used. The nurse will determine if the client has an impairment, such as visual problems. Because this is a possible symptom of a stroke, the HCA care plan should reflect any special considerations for communication.

Hearing Impairments

The hearing impaired client presents a special situation for the HCA. The following communication techniques have been broken down into supportive (those that improve the communication process) and nonsupportive (those techniques that make the situation worse) in working with clients who have hearing impairments.

Supportive communication techniques include:

1. Speaking clearly, slowly, in good lighting, and directly facing the hearing impaired client (Figure 11–8).

2. Being sure to get the client's attention before speaking. Do not start to speak abruptly.

3. Lowering the tone of your voice. Telephone bells, doorbells, horns, and emergency alarms should be toned down also.

4. Repeating what is said, using different words whenever it becomes necessary.

5. Knowing in which ear the client has better hearing, and speaking to that side.

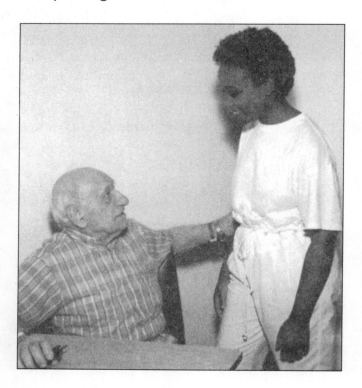

Figure 11–8 Face the hearing-impaired client directly and speak slowly and distinctly.

6. Recognizing that hearing declines as a normal aspect of aging. Convey this understanding through a supportive attitude.

7. Helping family members or those who work with older clients become better speakers by pointing out helpful speech habits such as those listed above.

Nonsupportive communication techniques include:

1. Shouting, which increases nonintelligible sounds and grossly distorts what the client hears.

2. Background noise, such as traffic or many persons talking at once.

3. Speaking too softly, running words together, or looking away from the hearing-impaired client while speaking.

4. Nonsupportive behaviors that interfere with lip reading.
   - exaggerated or distorted speech movements by persons trying to help the lip reader
   - speech that is too rapid
   - poor lighting on the speaker's face
   - mustaches that cover the lips
   - anything that covers the speaker's mouth such as cigars, pencils, fingers, food, or gum.

Visual Impairments

Working with clients who have visual impairments is a special situation that requires good communication techniques geared for that particular situation. The following are some guidelines for such a situation.

1. If the client has glasses, make sure they are clean and that he or she wears them. Also make sure that glasses are in good repair and fit correctly.

2. Provide adequate lighting at all times. Pools of bright light among darkened areas or variations in light intensity should be avoided.

3. Reduce glare by avoiding shiny surfaces, waxed floors, and exposed light bulbs. Have shades or sheer curtains at windows to reduce glare.

4. Brightly colored rims on dishes reduce spills.

5. Sharply contrasting colors for doors, bedspreads, floors, and walls help clients find their way and reduce accidents.

6. Large print newspapers, magazines, and books should be provided.

7. Refer to positions on the face of a clock to help the client locate items on a dinner plate or tray.

8. Clients with decreased peripheral vision may not see people or items sitting beside them.

9. Black telephones with white numerals are easier to see. Telephones with large numbers and letters on the dial are available.

10. Do not move personal belongings or furniture without the client's knowledge.

11. Consistently use sensory stimulation of sound, touch, and smell.

12. Use large clocks, clocks that chime, and radios to keep the client oriented to time.

13. Obtain talking books and other low-vision AIDS.

14. Numerals on doors and dials (such as a stove) should be large and distinct enough for clients with visual impairments to see or feel.

15. Magnifying glasses can be used

16. Give simple instructions and explanations for anything you plan to do, such as moving the client.

17. Sunglasses, sunvisors, caps, or hats with brims may help on rainy days or when there is snow.

Speaking Impairments (Aphasia)

Communicating with clients who have difficulty speaking (aphasia) creates another health care challenge. Clients who have had strokes are slow to regain their speaking abilities and require increased patience on the part of the HCA. Communication boards may be used to communicate with clients with aphasia (Figure 11–9). Some important principles to remember in this situation include:

1. Reducing your rate of speaking by prolonging the pauses between words and phrases when helping a client who is learning to speak.

2. Speaking in a normal tone of voice, emphasizing the main ideas, and using gestures to help clarify meanings.

3. Asking questions that can be answered with "yes" or "no" when requiring reliable information. For example, if the HCA wants to know what the client drank at dinner, ask "Did you have milk?" instead of "Did you have milk, coffee, or tea?"

4. Not supplying an anticipated word unless the client requests it because aphasia frequently causes a client frustration and embarrassment.

5. Not talking about a client in his or her presence. It is rude and can be discouraging to the client. Aphasic clients, espe-

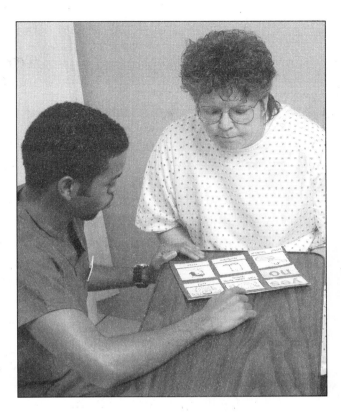

Figure 11–9 Communication boards or picture books may be used to communicate with patients with aphasia.

cially, may understand but be unable to express their thoughts and feelings.

6. Accepting errors and understanding that speech and language improve with time and proper training.

7. Never speaking to adult clients as though they were children. Doing so creates hurt feelings that could lead to frustration and depression, or feelings of resentment against the speaker. Adult clients, regardless of their abilities, are not children and do not deserve to be treated as such.

8. Not attempting to continue tasks that are frustrating to the client for long periods of time. Aphasic clients have a reduced ability to attend to activities for long periods of time and tire quickly. Arrange for short periods of activity and seek improvement in small steps so that some successes are achieved at each session.

9. Discouraging clients from remaining alone all day. Whenever possible, provide clients with opportunities for interacting with others in order for them to see that they are accepted and can enjoy life despite their aphasic difficulties.

10. Writing down what is to be conveyed if the accuracy of a message is critical, or if reinforcement of verbal and nonverbal communication is desired.

11. Giving positive reinforcement—both verbal and nonverbal—of the client's progress.

The ultimate goal in communication with home care clients is to provide the best ongoing care as possible. Sometimes this means making changes in care based on the information the HCA sees and hears. The information might simply help provide better care or serve a need to change the care plan. If the changes are serious enough, the supervisor will speak to the doctor to reevaluate the orders.

STRESSES ON THE CLIENT

Factors that the HCA should be aware of that can cause stress to the client who has had a stroke and may influence his or her recovery include:

- disturbance in sleep
- loss of friends
- loneliness
- fear of illness
- loss of a job
- decreasing eyesight
- fear of illness
- loss of mental abilities
- fear of impending death
- economic losses and concerns
- loss of driver's license
- fear of hospitalization
- illness of significant other
- feelings of dependency
- wish for more family visits
- less ability to care for oneself
- death of family member or close friend
- use of assistive devices
- loss of prior social or recreational activities
- regrets
- missing family members

CONFIDENTIALITY

confidentiality not taking the client's personal information outside the workplace

Confidentiality means that information about the client and family is personal and should not be repeated to persons outside of the workplace. The HCA must follow the basic guidelines for confidentiality:

Helpful Hint: Neighbors and friends are very curious about clients and their private lives. Be courteous but do not give personal information to other persons.

cultures behavior patterns or lifestyles of a particular race, nation, or group of people

1. Discuss the client's medical and personal facts only with the health care team.
2. It is the physician's responsibility and duty to tell the client medical information.
3. Do not discuss co-workers or workplace problems with peers or family; go to the supervisor (Figure 11–10).

HCA BEHAVIORS AND ATTITUDES

HCAs also come from many **cultures** and backgrounds. Each HCA brings his or her ethics or code of behavior to the home which is his or her workplace. These include:

- honesty with peers and clients
- respect of the home as a guest
- acceptance of differences in families
- reporting abuse
- caring for yourself and your appearance
- knowing and respecting the client's rights
- keeping a cheerful and positive attitude
- being dependable and on time
- never leaving the workplace with work unfinished
- not accepting tips or gifts
- knowing the HCAs rights
  Positive attitudes that reflect HCAs of the highest level include:
- being cheerful at tasks
- smiling during visits
- being happy to do extras
- having pride in appearance
- following directions well
- being empathetic to the client

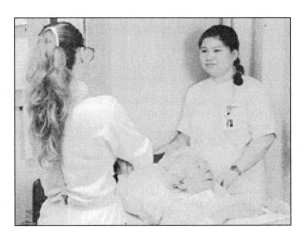

Figure 11–10 HCAs should not discuss personal activities in the presence of the client or family.

disability a permanent condition that causes physical or mental handicaps or weakness

psychosocial involving both psychological and social factors

- praising even small client participation
- leaving personal problems at home

Clients who have had a stroke are often weakened and disabled. These clients require an extra measure of consideration and care. A **disability** is a permanent condition that causes a physical or mental handicap or weakness caused by an accident, birth problem, or illness. Family responses to disabilities vary depending on the dynamics previously discussed. Client responses to disabilities also vary depending on that person's age, **psychosocial** background, the degree of the disability, economic factors, the family involvement and attitude, and the client's needs level. Some negative responses the HCA should recognize in client/ family to disabilities are anger, denial, withdrawal, and abuse.

Clients who have had a stroke should be given the opportunity to live at the highest level of self-care and self-respect, and in a safe and healthy environment.

SUMMARY

The physical care of the client recovering from a CVA is very important, but the psychosocial aspects are equally vital to his or her well-being. The health caregivers of today are aware that only caring for one part of a person's body leaves the rest of the person's needs unmet. Human beings have a mind, body, and spirit connection, and each affects the wellness of the other. The educated aide will look at all three aspects of each client and consider them equally important in the recovery process. This is best accomplished by considering the client an individual, with a unique cultural background and a set of needs exactly like no other person in the world. If the client is disabled or dying, these factors should be carefully considered when treating the whole person.

REVIEW QUESTIONS

1. List four barriers to the relationship between the HCA and the client/family.

   a.

   b.

   c.

   d.

2. Multicultural differences may occur in which area?

   a. race

   b. religion

   c. language

   d. diet

   e. all of the above

3. Which of the following is *not* an example of human physical needs?

   a. food

   b. water

   c. love

   d. rest

4. Which is *not* a psychological need?

   a. safety

   b. affection

   c. trust

   d. dignity

5. Which of the following is not an example of a factor contributing to differences in families that may affect the client?

   a. language

   b. technology

   c. cultures

   d. baby boomers

6. True or False? The HCA's acceptance of differences is important in the relationship with the client.

7. True or False? The HCA may discuss medical information with the family.

8. True or False? Anger is a typical client response to a disability or approaching death.

9. True or False? Decreasing numbers of friends is a source of stress for the client.

10. True or False? The client who has had a stroke does not feel stressed or concerned about increasing dependency on others.

11. True or False? Touch can be an effective means of communication.

12. True or False? If the client and/or family wish to teach the HCA some cultural phrases, the HCA should refuse.

13. Unscramble the following key term from the chapter: smipienmatr _____

Glossary

abuse inflicting physical or mental pain or injury on another person

activities of daily living tasks performed each day, such as toileting, bathing, dressing, feeding, grooming, homemaking, and other activities

adaptive equipment assists the client with ADLs

advocate a supporter; one who looks out for the safety and well-being of the client

amputation the surgical removal of all or part of a limb, usually the lower extremities above or below the knee

anticoagulant a medication that prevents or inhibits the clotting of blood

aphasia loss of language or speech

arterial sclerosis a build-up of cholesterol in the arteries

arthritis an inflammation or problem of the joint causing pain and limitation of movement of the joint

asepsis absence of pathogens

aspiration the inhalation of food or fluids into the lungs

atrophy muscle decreasing in size

autonomic nervous system that part of the nervous system which controls involuntary actions, and consists of the sympathetic and parasympathetic nervous systems

biofeedback a technique used to make involuntary actions of the body visible to the senses so as to make them voluntary

bladder training training to restore the client's ability to control urination

body mechanics correct and safe use of the body for work

bowel training training to restore the client's ability to control bowel movements

care plan a plan instituted by the nurse or physician which contains the goals, instructions, and specific orders for a sick or injured client

case conference meeting of all members of the health care team to analyze the client's case

case manager coordination; person in charge of the care of a specific client

central nervous system that part of the nervous system that consists of the brain and spinal cord which coordinates the activity of the entire system by interpreting incoming sensory impulses and sending out corresponding motor impulses

cerebral arteries any of the large vessels which carry oxygen to the cerebrum

cognitive loss loss associated with thinking or reasoning

compensate find an alternate way of completing a task

compliance the acceptance of medical instructions and medications by the client

confidentiality not taking the client's personal information outside the workplace

confused uncertain or unclear mentally

contracture when muscle tissue draws together or shortens because of spasm or paralysis (can be permanent or temporary)

cooperation common effort

coordination smooth interaction by all members of the team toward a common c goal

culture behavior patterns or lifestyles of a particular race, nation, or group of people

cerebral vascular accident or CVA (stroke) a disorder in which oxygenated blood flow to parts of the brain are blocked caused by a hemorrhage, thrombus, embolus, or arterial sclerosis

decubitus ulcers skin breakdown over body areas due to pressure or friction

deformities physical distortion of a body part

disability a permanent condition that causes physical or mental handicaps or weakness

disoriented confusion in the sense of identity or location

distractions activities or techniques to change the client's focus from his or her pain

documentation the written account of care given

education plan the day-to-day organization and process of the client/family teaching prepared by the nurse

elimination the process of ridding liquid waste from the body; urination

empower to authorize or strongly encourage another person

exercise equipment improves strength and mobility of the client

expected outcomes the hoped-for results of short and long-term goals

exploitation to use selfishly or unethically

family dynamics how the family interacts

flaccid lacking normal firmness or stiffness

flammable able to catch fire

functional limitations the client's level of ambulation and activity

gait training teaching the client the proper gait (walk) with assistive devices

goal purpose or objective to work toward

HCA care plan plan the HCA follows which is created by the nurse and updated every two weeks

hemiparesis muscle spasms or weakness

hemiplegia paralysis on one side of the body

hip disorders arthritis, hip fractures, and hip surgeries

home maintenance keeping the home a safe and healthy environment

holistic caring model care based on the belief that humans should be cared for as whole persons

hypertension high blood pressure

impairments disabilities caused by accident or illness

incontinence the inability to control bladder or bowel function

infection germs enter the body and cause disease

Interdisciplinary two or more disciplines working together

intervention any measure which modifies treatment or alters the course of a disease

involuntary muscles muscles that receive messages from the nervous system but work automatically without the person having to be aware

medical social worker (MSW) deals with spiritual, economic, and psychosocial problems

mobility ability to move or be moved

motivation act of encouraging another person to action

motivator a person who encourages another

multidiscipline various medical disciplines which make up a team to assist a particular client

neurons any of the cells of the nervous system, also called nerve cells

nursing care plan plan the nurse follows (nursing diagnoses) and the long- and short-term goals to solve patient problems

nursing diagnoses the specific issues in a client's recovery that are solely the responsibility of the nurse

occupation how the client is occupied in day-to-day living activities

occupational therapist (OT) assists in restoring muscle coordination and strength by increasing the client's activity and independence

oxygen (O_2) therapy administering oxygen by means of a cannula, mask, or nasal catheter

pain management pain control through techniques to reduce discomfort

paraplegic a client whose lower part of the body is paralyzed

pathogen disease-causing microorganisms

payors of home care Medicare, HMOs, or any insurance company that covers the client's health care expenses

peripheral nervous system that part of the nervous system which consists of cranial nerves, spinal nerves, and the autonomic nervous system

personal care devices special equipment designed to encourage self-care

physical therapist uses exercises and treatments to increase mobility

personal protective equipment (PPE) devices which form a barrier between health care workers and an infectious environment

psychosocial human interaction

PT plan of care care plan specific to PT care and treatments

quadriplegic a client paralyzed from the neck down

range of motion (ROM) exercises which move each muscle and joint through a full range of motion

rehabilitation center outpatient PT when large equipment is needed

rehabilitation equipment helps the client recover or improve activity

reinforce strengthen or support

respiratory therapist (RT) restores the best level of breathing through breathing exercises

retaliation repayment in kind; usually revenge

safe environment an environment in which a person has a very low risk of illness or injury

safety devices devices used to prevent accident or injury to a sick or disabled client

self-esteem self respect; self-image

semiprone position lying in bed with head and shoulders elevated

signs client changes that can be seen, felt, heard or smelt

spasm an involuntary movement of muscle

speech therapist (ST) assists in speech and communication improvement

standard precautions new guidelines which replace the original universal precautions of infection control

supportive devices protect the client from falling when ambulating

symptoms client's stated complaints

TENS unit electrical stimulation of nerves to reduce pain

voluntary muscles movement is controlled by the conscious brain

weight bearing amount of body weight placed on a hip or leg

window period the period of time in which a treatment or medical procedure will be of benefit to a client

Index

Page numbers followed by an f denote figures and numbers followed by a t denote tables.